KB152067

Anatomical Liver Resection
: Toward Tailored Surgery

HEE JUNG WANG

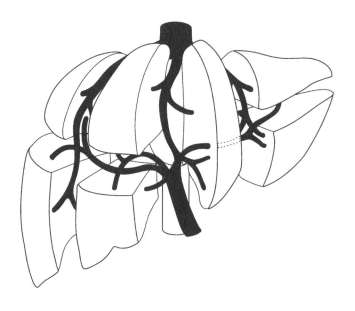

KOONJA

Anatomical Liver Resection
: Toward Tailored Surgery

1st Print : 2020-08-13
1st Publication : 2020-08-28

Author : Hee Jung Wang
Planner : Hee Sung Jang
Editor : Kyung Eun Lee
Designer : Ran Hee Yang
Illustrator : Kyung Yeol Kim
Publishing House : Koonja Publishing, Inc.
       Registration No. 4-139 (June 24, 1991)
       Paju Publishing Complex, 338, Hoedong-gil (474-1 Seopae-dong),
       Paju-si, Gyeonggi-do, South Korea (10881)
       Tel: (82)-31-943-1888 Fax: (82)-31-955-9545
       Web: www.koonja.co.kr

* Damaged copies will be replaced.
* The seal has been omitted under agreement with the authors.

ISBN   979-11-5955-596-1
USD $41.99

I dedicate this book to our gracious God who led the Department of Hepatobiliary Surgery, Ajou University Hospital and myself for the past twenty-five years until today.

Preface

I was honorably invited to speak in front of the audience for one hour at the workshop for hepatobiliary-pancreas surgeons with the title "Liver Surgery: Ajou University Style" on July 6th, 2019, a year before my retirement. Taken this opportunity, I spoke about the liver surgery that has been performed and the surgical philosophy we are pursuing. With this in mind, I thought that it would be meaningful to record in detail, the procedures carried out at Ajou University Hospital. On the other hand, it has been 25 years since I started working at the Department of Hepatobiliary Surgery in this institution, and it is now time to leave my work behind for young surgeons to take over and leap forward for future decades to come. The idea of leaving is the starting point for writing this book.

Department of Surgery, Ajou University has been performing over three thousand liver operations since the hospital's opening in year 1994, and I had put much effort on teaching young surgeons that the anatomical liver resection (AR) within the limits of liver function must be the standard treatment of choice as I was taught likewise. However, AR was not possible in all cases due to variations in intrahepatic anatomy when dealing with right-side liver resection. In such cases, fissural approach was preferred among the Glissonean approaches to overcome difficulties. Pietro Majno and colleagues recently pointed out that Couinaud's scheme of liver anatomy is rather over-simplified, and suggested that a tailored surgery according to the 3D image analysis is required. By introducing 3D synapse (Fujifilm) to our institution in 2016, I tried to raise the success rate of AR by performing so-called tailored procedures, according to the intuitive reconstruction image of the intrahepatic

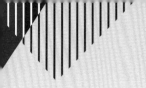

vasculature which was obtained prior to the surgery. In this book I will share my experience.

I would like to express my gratitude to professor Cho, Sung-won, first head of Liver Center and to all colleagues in the department of Hepatology, Radiology, Anesthesiology and Critical Care Medicine. I am, also, grateful to the surgeons, nurses in operation room and intensive care unit, coordinators and physician assistants (PAs) who had put enormous amount of effort to caregiving.

Lastly, I am deeply grateful to professor Hong, Sung Yeon for his painstaking and tremendous translation work, to professor Hu, XuGuang for editing videos, and to professor Yoon, Duk Yong for the statistical analysis to make a publication of this book. The publisher, especially Ms. Lee, Kyung Eun, has also made a significant contribution to this book.

December 2019
Wang, Hee Jung

Table of contents

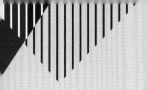

Contents of CD

Transfissural/Glissonean approaches of Hepatectomy

Anatomical Liver Resection
: Toward Tailored Surgery

1

Introduction

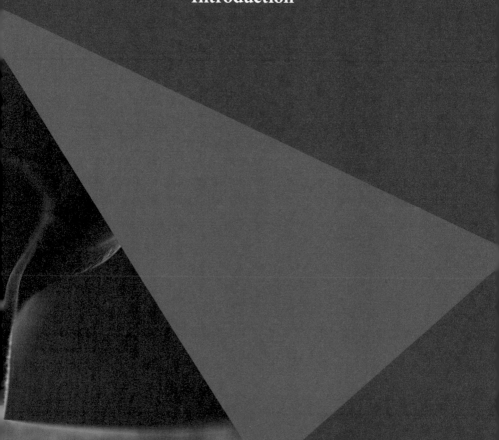

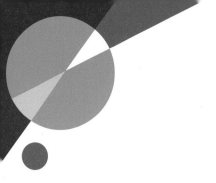

Introduction

There was no description of liver surgery in the textbook before 1950. All available were a handful of case reports. In the 1950s and 1960s, Tong That Tung, Claude de Couinaud and Henry Bismuth began to come up with the theories and modern concepts of liver anatomy and liver resection. This fashion was followed by Masatoshi Makuuchi, Bernard Launois, Leslie H. Blumgart and Ken Takasaki who continued to develop surgical technique of liver surgery in their own continent; Asia, Europe and America. **(Figure 1)** During this period,

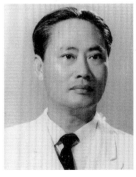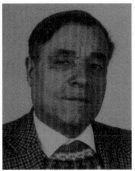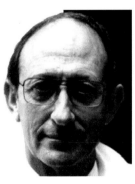

| Tong That Tung | Claude de Couinaud | Henri Bismuth |

• **Figure 1** **Pioneers in modern concepts and techniques of liver surgery.**

there were subtle dissimilarities on the view of liver anatomy and techniques of liver resection for each institution in their nations, until the year 2000, the terms of liver anatomy and liver surgery were unified at the International Hepato-Pancreato-Biliary Association (IHPBA) congress. It took 50 years for this achievement to be made.

Recently, 3-dimentional depiction of liver anatomy has become possible. With the aid of this new technology, Pietro Majno and colleagues proposed a novel interpretation of liver anatomy as "1-2-20 concept" in 2014. It is based on their observation of the intrahepatic vasculature such that the hepatic inflow or portal vein gives three 1st order branches; left, right anterior and right posterior; and further divides into random 2nd order branches, 9 to 44 in number (mean=20) rather than eight segmental branches, as conventional Couinaud's model describes. Majno's model is somewhat parallel to Takasaki's "cone unit" scheme. The notorious H. Bismuth supported this view of liver anatomy and wrote in his editorial: "The paper by Majno et al. makes the interesting proposal that we should retain the Couinaud's division of the liver into 8 segments but that we should be ready to break free from it when, as radiologists and surgeons, we perform the complex procedures that the modern treatment of surgical liver disease requires." He, also, quoted Julien Benda's line: "The human race wants simple ideas, but reality is complicated", suggesting adaptation to the anatomical complexity and a tailored surgical approach are the call of the times, and we must embrace the change.

Against this backdrop, I began this writing to summarize and record in detail as to the novel view on liver anatomy in the era of 3D imaging of intrahepatic vasculature. First, I will start by looking back past 25 years of my experience of liver resection under Couinaud's dogma, and I will, then, discuss the importance and usefulness of reviewing the 3D image prior to the surgery. However, I would like to point out that all of the contents of this book on liver anatomy and liver resection were thoroughly loyal to the Couinaud's theory.

Anatomical Liver Resection
: Toward Tailored Surgery

2

Clinical anatomy of the liver

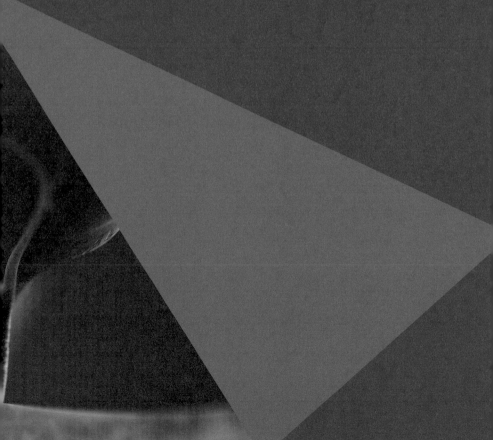

2
Clinical anatomy of the liver

Segmental anatomy of the liver was first described by Claude de Couinaud in 1950s, such that two intrahepatic vascular systems (portal and venous vasculature) divide the liver in 8 segments. The three 2nd order branches of Glisson pedicles (portal vein, hepatic artery and bile duct tree) and three outflow vessels (right, middle and left hepatic veins) lie within the liver in the shape of fingers of two hands interlocked. The vascular perfusion territories border one another by the plane formed by the opponent vascular system. Glisson pedicle is synonymous to the portal pedicle beyond 2nd order branch level, for the reference.

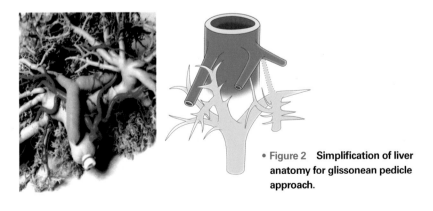

• **Figure 2 Simplification of liver anatomy for glissonean pedicle approach.**

There are three major anatomical knowledge to be mastered when applying the Glissonean approach to batch-process the three structures within the Glissonean sheath during liver resection. First, the vascular anatomy of the liver must be speculated in a simplified view. Hepatic inflow is regarded as the Glisson pedicle and the outflow as the hepatic veins. **(Figure 2)** The second is that there are, frequent variation of the branches of the portal vein, hepatic artery and bile duct crossing the boundary within the territories of first order branches **(Figure 3)**, whereas there is no variation of crossing the boundaries in the territories of 2nd order branches and Couinaud segmental branches. Therefore, the ligation of Glisson pedicle must be performed at the level of 2nd order branches or further when applying Glissonean approach during liver resection **(Figure 4)**. Third, Glissonean pedicles have a certain rules of variation within the liver

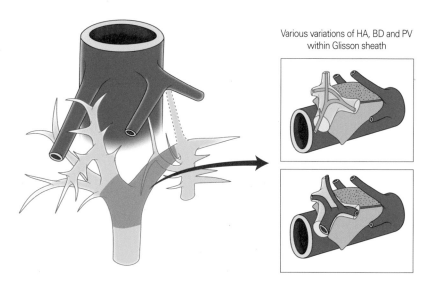

Various variations of HA, BD and PV within Glisson sheath

• Figure 3   **Anatomical variations of inflow structures in hilar pedicle. (Couinaud C, 1981)**

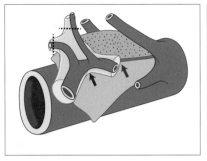 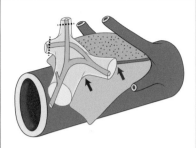

• Figure 4   Technique to avoid inadequate injuries in glissonean approach during right hepatectomy / left hepatectomy.

... Safe division level of Glisson pedicles in right hepatectomy

🡑 Safe division level of Glisson pedicle in left hepatectomy (🡑 potential inadequate injury)

parenchyma. Couinaud's segmental Glisson pedicles of the left lobe have variations only in number of segmental pedicles (**Figure 5**), and that of the right lobe might have variations in both number of pedicles and sliding of origins (**Figure 6**)[1].

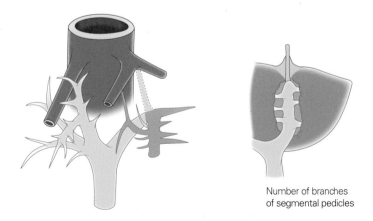

Number of branches
of segmental pedicles

• Figure 5   Anatomical Variations of intrahepatic Glisson pedicles in left liver. (only variation of number of branches of segmental pedicles (Couinaud C, 1981)

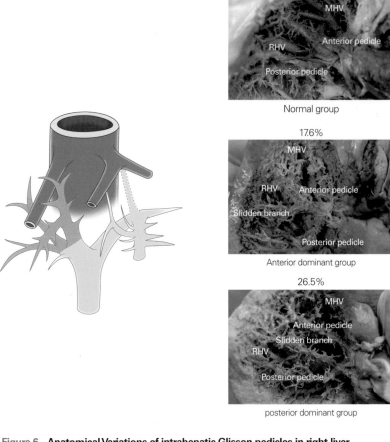

55.9%

MHV
Anterior pedicle
RHV
Posterior pedicle

Normal group

17.6%

MHV
RHV
Anterior pedicle
Slidden branch
Posterior pedicle

Anterior dominant group

26.5%

MHV
Anterior pedicle
Slidden branch
RHV
Posterior pedicle

posterior dominant group

• Figure 6　Anatomical Variations of intrahepatic Glisson pedicles in right liver.
(Variation of sliding of origin of segmental Pedicles)[1]

According to my experience in cadaver dissection, 55.9% of population had no sliding of origin type variation (normal type), 17.6% had terminal branches of right posterior sector (RPS) which were slidden from the right anterior sector (RAS) territory (anterior dominant type), and 26.5% had terminal branches of right anterior sector that was slidden from the posterior sector territory (posterior dominant type) **(Figure 6)**. How would this type of variation affect the Glissonean approach of liver resection? In case of the right anterior sectionectomy in the liver which is a posterior dominant type with small sliding branches, the ischemic demarcation after right anterior pedicle clamp can be seen at the left side of the right hepatic vein (RHV) so that RHV cannot be exposed at the transection plane. On the contrary, in anterior dominant variant liver, the ischemic demarcation is formed at the right side over the RHV. If the surgeons intends to retrieve the RHV, the dissection plane might trespass the RAS, leaving the non-perfused liver tissue at the dorsal portion of the RHV. Could this be defined as an anatomical resection (AR)? Strictly speaking, it is not an AR. Rather I would like to refer to this type of resection as "near-AR". In our statistics they are classified as ARs only if the variation is a small one and I had to leave a negligible amount of non-perfused liver parenchyma. When the sliding pedicle is significantly large, modifications in surgical technique should be made, which I will discuss in chapter 5 section 2.

3

Definition and necessity of the anatomical resection

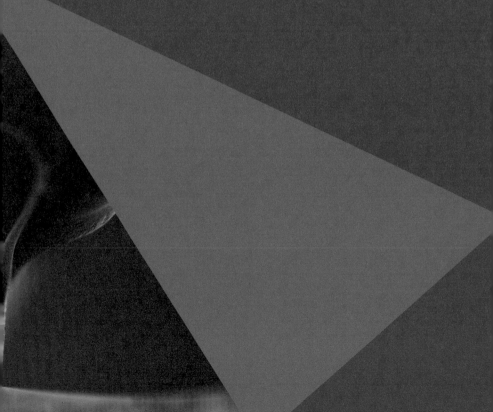

3

Definition and necessity of the anatomical resection

Hepatocellular carcinoma (HCC) initially receives blood flow from the hepatic artery and portal vein as in the liver parenchyma. As the tumor gradually grows, neovascularization from the hepatic artery forms into the tumor tissue, pushing the portal and hepatic veins to the periphery. As the pressure of the portal vein becomes lower than that of arterial inflow of the tumor, portal vein play a role as the outflow of the tumor. (Figure 7)[2, 3]. Miura et al. conducted a study on hemodynamics of human liver with HCC using 3D vascular reconstruction image by angio-CT and a software that utilizes region growing and fusion image technique. They found that the portal vein is mainly responsible for the outflow of HCCs with expanding growth pattern. (Figure 8).[4] With this knowledge in the background, Makuuchi et al. proposed a theory that partial liver resection for HCC requires resection of portal-perfusion area of tumor bearing parenchyma (Figure 9) and this is the theoretical background of the systematic hepatectomy. In other words, the definition of systematic liver resection (SR) is a term referred to as liver resection that removes the tumor-bearing portal territory confirmed by temporary clamping or dye-injection of the portal branch. (Figure 10)[5]. Based on Couinaud's theory, an AR refers to the liver resection, the territory of which corresponds to the inflow and outflow volume of portal vein and hepatic vein. A RAS, for example,

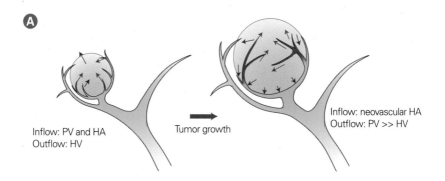

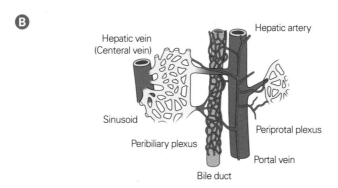

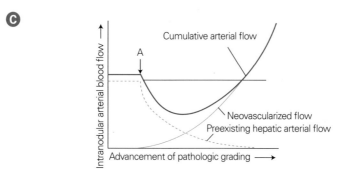

• Figure 7　Development of intratumoral blood flow in HCC. A. Changes of inflow and
outflow in HCC according to tumor growth. B. Intrahepatic vascular collaterals.[2]
C. Changes of inflow blood volume and kinds of inflow vessels.[3]

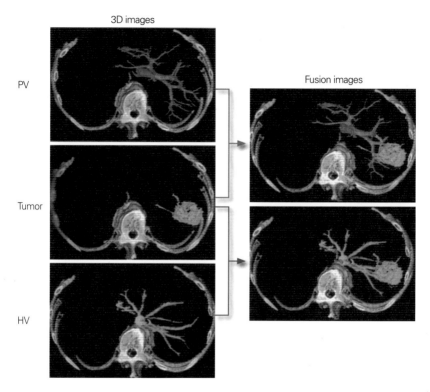

PV

Tumor

HV

3D images

Fusion images

• **Figure 8   Imaging study for the draining pathway of intratumoral outflow in HCC.**[4]

right anterior portal pedicle perfusion area, bordered by the planes formed by RHV and MHV is the resection area for AR.**(Figure 11)**[6] So, are AR and SR the same operation? Or is it another type of surgery? In the case of left and right hepatectomy, sectionectomies and segmentectomy 1, AR is identical to SR in most of the cases. However, AR and SR are not completely consistent in about 40%, when there is an anatomical variation of the sliding of origin pattern in the right hepatectomy **(Figure 6)**.[1] Therefore, not all but some Japanese surgeons such as Takasaki only admit that surgery, extent of which exceeds sectionctomy as an AR, and regard monosegmentectomies as non-AR. I will discuss this is detail in the next chapters.

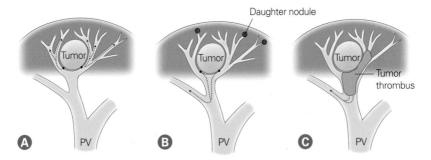

- **Figure 9** Rationale of systematic resection.[5] A possible form of intrahepatic extension of HCC: (A) An HCC invades nearby portal venous branches and tumor cells are carried to the periphery. (B) These cells form microscopic tumor thrombi and then intrahepatic metastases. (C) Tumor thrombi are a source of wider spread.

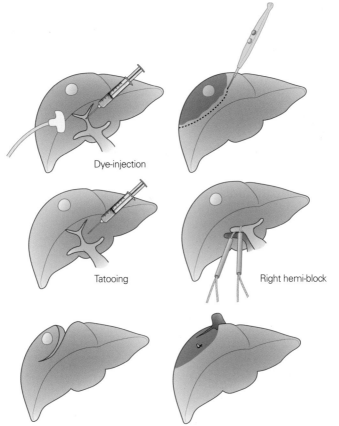

Dye-injection

Tatooing

Right hemi-block

- **Figure 10** Definition of systematic resection.[5] To remove the tumor bearing liver parenchyma which is discolored from dye-injection or clamping of specific inflow portal pedicle.

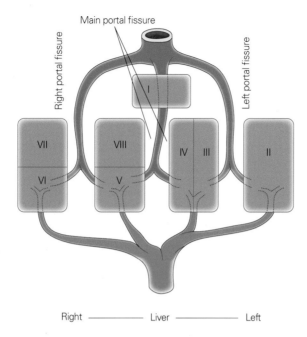

● Figure 11　Definition of anatomical resection.[6] The 4 portal sections are divided by 3 portal fissures. Three hepatic veins lie in the 3 portal fissures. When we do inflow oriented resection, we can always meet hepatic vein(s) on the resected margin.

4

Anatomical variations in intrahepatic vasculature and recent clinical approaches

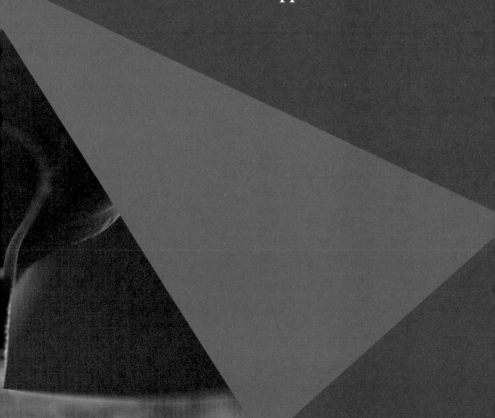

4

Anatomical variations in intrahepatic vasculature and recent clinical approaches

4.1
Research on the variation of right liver using 3D images

Couinaud's eight-segment scheme, despite its usefulness and simplicity, can serve as a dogma that divides liver in a man-made fashion. In general, liver has a constant first and second order inflow branches that divides the organ into two hemilivers and four sections which have watershed plane where the hepatic veins are located. However, this schema of anatomical description, renders or even preclude inflow-oriented anatomical liver resection as it neglects the variation of inflow vessels in terms of number of branches and sliding of their origins. In the next section, the variation of inflow of the right hemiliver by the present author's experience in cadaveric liver dissection and 3D image analysis is to be discussed.

Our institution adopted Synapse 3D (Fuji film) in 2016, and we analyzed the variation of third order inflow branches to the right anterior and posterior sections (RAS and RPS) in 96 liver donors from 2017 to 2018. The result showed that the portal pedicles to the RAS have 4 different branching types; A-D. A cranio-caudal type or type A is when the third order branch structure correspond to the Couinaud's segment 5 and 8 anatomy, and comprised 45.8% (44) of the cases. Ventral-dorsal type or type B (13, 13.5%) is responsible for the liver, segment 5 and 8 of which are supplied by two or more fourth order branches from a different third order branch. A radial type or type C (33, 34.4%) is when there are multiple usually more than 4 third order branches present. In this cases, segments 5 and 8 cannot be distinguished. In the slidden type or type D (6, 6.3%), the third or fourth order branches of the RAS and RPS trespasses to the other territories. **(Figure 12)**

The RPS, likewise, has four distinct anatomical entities. Type A is whereby the right posterior portal pedicle has a common trunk (a second order branch) and further gives its branches (two) to each segments 6 and 7, and comprised 34.4% (33cases). In type B, similarly, the right posterior section pedicles branch to each segments but in absence of a common trunk (14, 14.6%). The right posterior portal pedicle in type C runs through the liver parenchyma towards the segment 7 and gives multiple branches to segment 6. (43, 44.8%). Lastly, the type D is likewise of the type D of RAS variation. **(Figure 13)**

In conclusion, a strictly controlled anatomical resection of segments 7 and 8 can be performed in only 49% (A or B type of RPS variant) and 45.8% (A type of RAS variant) of all cases, respectively. However, given that 3D CT image reconstruction is available, a higher success rate of anatomical resection can be achieved by designing the resection plane according to the individual anatomy. Otherwise, a larger extent of liver resection or non-anatomical wedge resection must be selected in patients with variant anatomy. Further discussion on this matter is in chapter 8.

Type A: cranial-caudal type (49 cases, 46.2%)
The 3rd order portal branch of anterior portal pedicle have two or more branch and they go to the cranial-caudal direction.

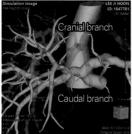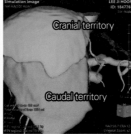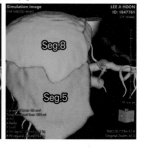

Type B: ventral-dorsal type (14 cases, 13.2%)
The 3rd order portal branch of anterior portal pedicle have two or more branch and they go to the ventral-dorsal direction.

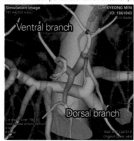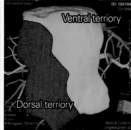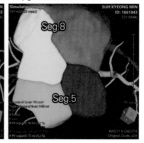

Type C: Radial type (37 cases, 34.9%)
The 3rd order portal branch of anterior portal pedicle have multiple branches and they go to the radial direction.

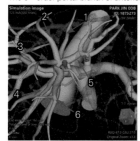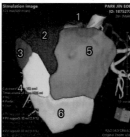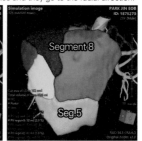

Type D: The right anterior Glission pedicles have slidden branch to/from posterior branch (6 cases, 5.7%)
branch of anterior portal pedicle comes from posterior portal pedicle.

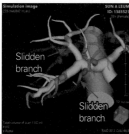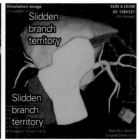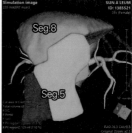

• Figure 12   Anatomical Variations of Anterior Sectional Pedicles
3D images using Synapse 3D (Fuji film) in 96 LDLT donor livers (Ajou Univ. 2017-2018)

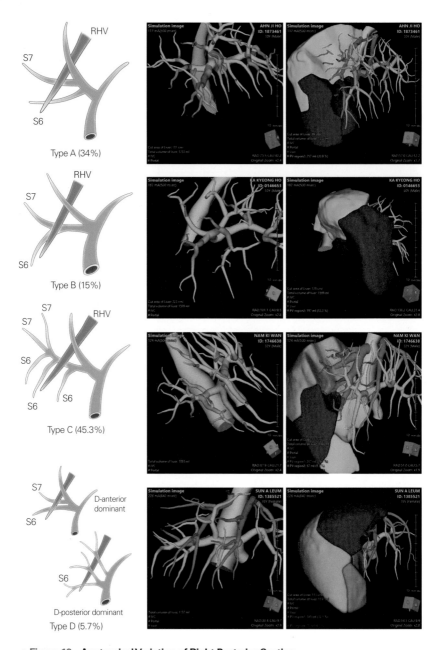

• **Figure 13** **Anatomical Variation of Right Posterior Section**

3D images using Synapse 3D (Fuji film) in 96 LDLT donor livers (Ajou Univ. 2017-2018)

4.2
Clinical approach according to the Pietro Majno's complexity of anatomy

P. Majno explained that the segmental anatomy of the liver has complexity in 3D image analysis, which can hardly be understood by a simple Couinaud's anatomy and suggested "1-2-20 concept". It is based on their observation of the intrahepatic vasculature such that the hepatic inflow or portal vein gives three 1st order branches; left, right anterior and right posterior; and further divides into random 2nd order branches, 9 to 44 in number (mean=20) rather than eight segmental branches, as conventional Couinaud's model describes. In analogy to Couinaud's 8 segment scheme, each segment must be supplied by single segmental Glissonean pedicles, but in real life, branching pattern is quite irregular and random. To facilitate communication among doctors, Glisson pedicle of the liver starts with one in the interrogating part, and two 1st order branches arise from it; right and left. The second order branches correspond to right anterior and posterior to the right lobe, and segment 2 branch and umbilical portion beyond Arantius duct to the left lobe. This architecture is constant in most cases, and the structure that form the boundaries or each territories are three hepatic veins. Therefore, "1-2-4-20" law is a more precise description. In other words, it's the 3rd order branches that are randomly arisen (Figure 14). Randomness in the context describes that there might be variation in number of branches in the left lobe and "sliding of origin" pattern variation along with variation of number of branches in the right lobe of the liver. Under the background of this understanding, I would like to discuss P Majno's three levels of complexity of intrahepatic vasculature (Figure 15). He reclaimed the actual portal vasculature is more complex than Couinaud's 8 segment structure and suggested three levels of complexity. First level is identical to Couinaud's 8 segment scheme serves as a common language between clinicians. This level views hepatic vasculature is composed of three hepatic veins and four 2nd order branches of portal pedicles. Second level is not a simplified or theoretical stage of anatomy, but rather is an anatomical level based on the actual branching pattern of Glissonean pedicles

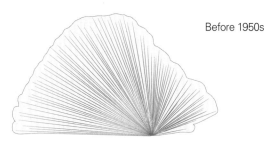

Before 1950s

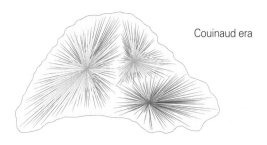

Couinaud era

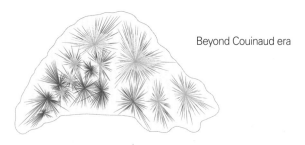

Beyond Couinaud era

• **Figure 14   Anatomical variation of the third order branches of portal pedicles**

This slide shows complexity of third order branches of portal pedicle by Professor Majno. He reported that the number of 3rd order branches are so much variable from 9 to 44, and not 8 of Couinaud anatomy. There is no rule in the branching pattern.

(Majno P et al. Anatomy of the liver: An outline with three level of complexity – A further step towards tailored territorial liver resection. J Hepatol 2014;60:654-662)[15]

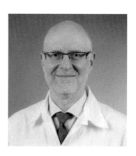

● Figure 15   Liver Anatomy: Three levels of complexity[15]

(Majno P et al. Anatomy of the liver: An outline with three level of complexity – A further step towards tailored territorial liver resection. J Hepatol 2014;60:654-662)

that allows surgeons to identify vascular structure by 3D image in modern liver surgery. By this understanding, tailored territorial liver resections have become possible. However, an approach independent of the Couinaud anatomy is required for this level of complexity. Finally, the third level of complexity of liver anatomy (academic level) is a step for anatomists based on the diversity and randomness of portal pedicle branching which allows us to understand the complexity of the vascular tree and segmental anatomy free from Couinaud's dogma; 1-2-20 or 1-2-4-20 concept sums up the complexity.

4.3
Effort on the tailored liver resection

A more delicate approach or tailored (individual anatomy-oriented) surgery has become possible nowadays, aided by 3D imaging and new surgical techniques. In the end, what is new here is the concept of preoperative simulation of liver resection and navigation during surgery. What I have experienced in the last three years is that preoperative simulation using Synapse 3D (Fuji Film, Tokyo) software by visualizing 3D structure of the intrahepatic vascular structure and by performing a mock surgery at the workstation **(Figures 16, 17)**. Moreover, navigation during the surgery is available. Recently, liver tumors are being discovered at their early stages and laparoscopic hepatic resection has gradually expanded. ICG fluorescent technique is used to depict the tumor and future remnant liver or resected liver **(Figures 18)**, and sometimes phantom of the liver is used to explain

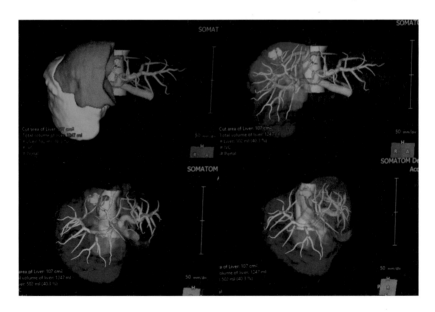

• Figure 16   **Preoperative simulation using 3D-imaging**

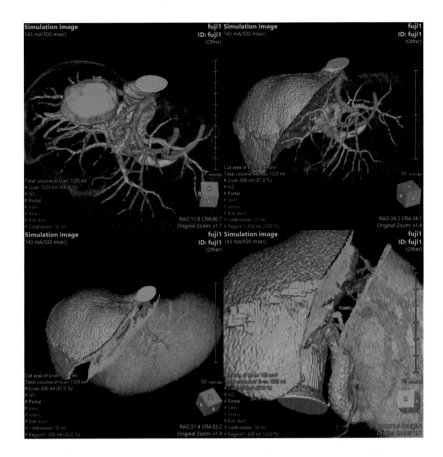

Simulation image
143 mA(500 msec)

fuji1 Simulation image
ID: fuji1 143 mA(500 msec)
(Other)

fuji1
ID: fuji1
(Other)

Cut area of liver 112 cm²
Total volume of liver: 1329 ml
Liver: 890 ml (67.0 %)
IVC
Portal
Vein
Artery
Bile duct
RAO:11.8 CRA:48.7 # Gallbladder: 58 ml
Original Zoom: x1.7 # Region1: 438 ml (33.0 %)

Total volume of liver: 1329 ml
Liver: 1329 ml (100.0 %)
IVC
Portal
Vein
Artery
Gallbladder: 58 ml

50 mm/div

RAO:34.3 CRA:34.1
Original Zoom: x1.4

Simulation image
143 mA(500 msec)

fuji1 Simulation image
ID: fuji1 143 mA(500 msec)
(Other)

fuji1
ID: fuji1
(Other)

Cut area of Liver: 112 cm²
Total volume of liver: 1329 ml
Liver: 890 ml (67.0 %)
IVC
Portal
Vein
Artery
Bile duct
Gallbladder: 58 ml
Region1: 438 ml (33.0 %)

RAO:51.4 CRA:53.2
Original Zoom: x1.3

• Figure 17   Preoperative procedural simulation using 3D-imaging

disease and its surgery to patient's family or use it as the intraoperative navigation.**(Figure 19, 20)** I believe that preoperative 3D imaging is essential for ensuring accuracy in all such procedures. The specific examples are shown in chapter 8.

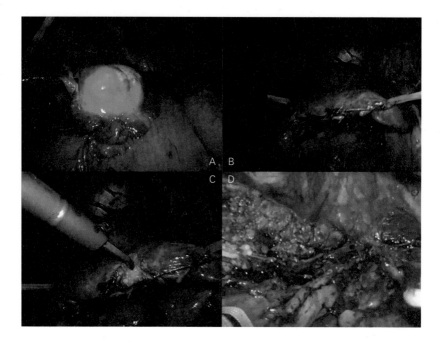

• **Figure 18　ICG fluorescent navigation surgery. This is ICG fluorescent finding of HCC.**

It was made by preoperative iv infusion of ICG (0.5mg/kg) 2 days before hepatectomy. (A)
And this picture is ICG fluorescent finding of future remnant liver, and it was made by intraoperative
iv infusion of ICG (0.01 mg/kg) after division of left portal pedicle. (B)
Parenchymal dissection was started under the intermittent ICG fluororescent navigation. (C) This is
operative field after left hemihepatectomy. (D)

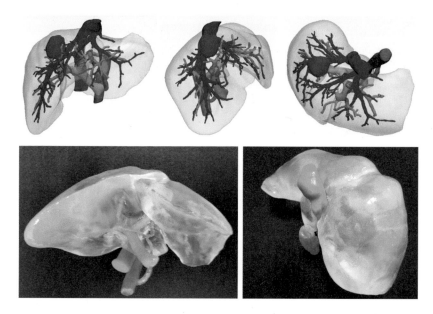

• Figure 19   Phantom of the liver made from 3D printing

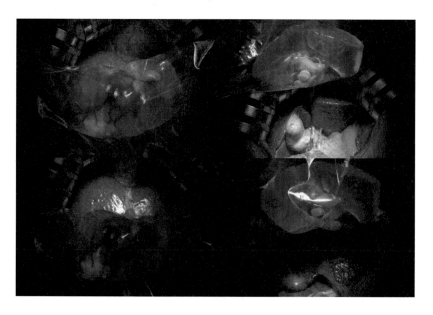

• Figure 20   Intraoperative navigation using phantom of the liver

Anatomical Liver Resection
: Toward Tailored Surgery

5

Oncological aspect of anatomical resection

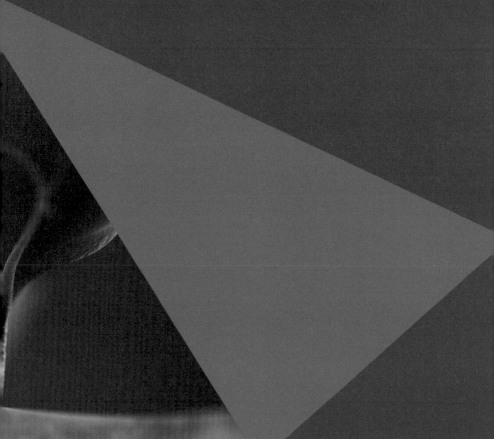

5

Oncological aspect of anatomical resection

5.1
Controversy between anatomical and non-anatomical resection

Despite Makuuchi's opinion, it is still a controversy whether AR influences postoperative prognosis of liver cancer. Most liver surgeons believe that systematic resection (SR, ie. AR) is superior to the non-AR in treating early HCCs and try to apply AR in every cases possible. Moreover, a non-AR tends to leave more de-vascularized tissue by injuring portal vasculature in the remnant liver. Since more than 60% of the HCC patients are accompanied by liver cirrhosis, this necrotic tissue after liver resection is likely to act as a metabolic burden to recover residual liver function, and may lead to post-hepatectomy liver failure. However, residual liver function after liver resection may limit the resection volume, and therefore, surgeons are frequently obliged to perform a non-anatomical limited resection. According to a multicenter questionnaire in 10 university hospitals in South Korea, surgeons replied that they have performed 73.9% of AR in small HCC, among which 34.4% were major resections and 65.6% were limited minor resections. They, also, reported there was no difference in cumulative survival and disease-free survival between AR and non-AR.[10] Now, the questions are: What are the criteria for an AR? To what extent should we call them ARs? In the survey, each surgeon was left to subjective judgment. There is no objective judgment to use in the current situation. In my opinion, the AR rate was overestimated. The criteria for AR is too generous. The more generous this standard is, the more likely it is that the oncological significance of the AR is faded.

5.2
Outcomes of anatomical resection in previous literature

Among the papers related to liver resection for HCC that have been reported in the literature in the past decade, there are 38 papers on whether there is a difference in the prognosis after AR compared to non-AR. Among them, 7 with good design were reviewed. There are a similar number of articles that state there was no difference from articles which pointed AR was superior to non-AR, and some reported AR produced better oncologic outcome in patients with HCC larger than 2cm or 2 to 5cm in diameter. **(Table 1)**[7-9] In order to get answer to this controversy, two meta-analysis papers were published on this subject in 2011. They, also, showed contradicting results as to that AR and non-AR differed in terms of cumulative and disease-free survival rates. The prognosis after surgery (AR vs. non-AR) is yet to be concluded. **(Table 2,3)**[7,8]

Table 1 Review of the literature on AR vs. NAR for HCC in the last decade.[7-9]

Paper	Patients		mortality(%)	5-year survival	Conclusion
Hasegawa (2005)	AR	156	0	66	AR
	NAR	54	0	35	
Kaibori (2006)	AR	34	2.9	52.7	NAR
	NAR	213	1.9	46.2	
Regimbeau (2002)	AR	30	7	54	AR
	NAR	34	6	35	
Tanaka (2008)	AR	83	0	54	NAR
	NAR	42	0	61	
Wakai (2007)	AR	95	2	67	AR if>2cm
	NAR	63	6	59	
Yamazaki (2010)	AR	111	1.8	71	AR if>2cm
	NAR	98	0	48	
Eguchi (2008)	AR	2267	0.7	65.5	AR if 2-5cm
	NAR	3514	0.8	62.4	

Table 2 Two papers of meta-analysis for comparison of oncologic outcome between anatomical resection and non-anatomical resection for HCC in 2011.[7,8]

There are conflicting results between two meta-analysis in overall survival

Zhou Y

Study or sub-category	AR group n/N	NAR group n/N	OR (random) 95% CI	Weight %	OR (random) 95 % CI
Yamamoto 2001	60/90	64/114		8.52	1.56 [0.88, 2.77]
Regimbeau 2002	16/30	12/34		5.80	2.10 [0.77, 5.72]
Hasegawa 2005	103/156	19/54		8.01	3.58 [1.87, 6.85]
Kaibori 2006	18/34	114/213		7.50	0.98 [0.47, 2.02]
Cho 2007	65/99	34/69		8.15	1.97 [1.05, 3.69]
Wakai 2007	67/95	37/63		7.94	1.45 [0.75, 2.81]
Yamashita 2007	152/201	89/120		8.88	1.08 [0.64, 1.82]
Nanashima 2008	27/49	42/64		7.25	0.64 [0.30, 1.38]
Tanaka 2008	45/83	26/42		7.28	0.73 [0.34, 1.55]
Ueno 2008	35/52	36/64		7.26	1.60 [0.75, 3.43]
Kamiyama 2010	148/169	86/153		8.63	5.49 [3.14, 9.59]
Kang 2010	67/146	9/21		6.26	1.13 [0.45, 2.85]
Yamazaki 2010	79/111	47/98		8.54	2.68 [1.51, 4.74]
Total (95% CI)	1315	1109		100.00	1.63 [1.15, 2.32]

Total events: 879 (AR group), 615 (NAR group)
Test for heterogeneity: $\chi 2 = 42.10$, df = 12 (p<0.0001), I^2=71.5%
Test for overall effect: Z = 2.74 (p = 0.006)

0.1 0.2 0.5 1 2 5 10

Favours AR group   Favours NAR group

Chen J

Study or sub-category	AR n/N	NAR n/N	OR (random) 95% CI	Weight %	OR (random) 95 % CI
Capussotti 2005	56/164	21/52		12.79	0.77 [0.40, 1.45]
Hasegawa 2005	103/156	19/54		12.64	3.58 [1.87, 6.85]
Kaibori 2006	18/34	114/213		11.41	0.98 [0.47, 2.02]
Regimbeau2002	16/30	12/34		7.86	2.10 [0.77, 5.72]
Tanaka 2008	45/83	26/42		10.92	0.73 [0.34, 1.55]
Ueno 2008	34/52	35/64		10.97	1.57 [0.74, 3.33]
Wakai 2006	64/95	37/63		12.47	1.45 [0.75, 2.81]
Yamashitta 2007	153/201	89/120		14.97	1.11 [0.66, 1.87]
Ziparo 2002	7/18	10/28		5.98	1.15 [0.34, 3.89]
Total (95% CI)	833	670		100.00	1.31 [0.92, 1.85]

Total events: 496 (AR), 363 (NAR)
Test for heterogeneity: Chi² = 16.41, df = 8 (p=0.04), I² = 51.2%
Test for overall effect: Z = 1.50 (p = 0.013)

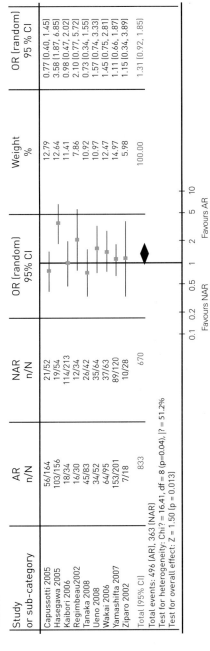

0.1 0.2   0.5   1   2   5   10

Favours NAR   Favours AR

Table 3 Two papers of meta-analysis for comparison of oncologic outcome between anatomical resection and non-anatomical resection for HCC in 2011.[7,8]

There are conflicting results between two meta-analysis in recurrence free survival

Zhou Y

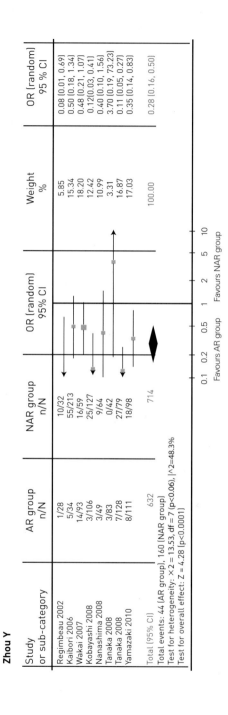

Study or sub-category	AR group n/N	NAR group n/N	OR (random) 95% CI	Weight %	OR (random) 95% CI
Regimbeau 2002	1/28	10/32		5.85	0.08 [0.01, 0.69]
Kaibori 2006	5/34	55/213		15.34	0.50 [0.18, 1.34]
Wakai 2007	14/93	16/59		18.20	0.48 [0.21, 1.07]
Kobayashi 2008	3/106	25/127		12.42	0.12 [0.03, 0.41]
Nanashima 2008	3/49	9/64		10.99	0.40 [0.10, 1.56]
Tanaka 2008	3/83	0/42		3.31	3.70 [0.19, 73.23]
Tanaka 2008	7/128	27/79		16.87	0.11 [0.05, 0.27]
Yamazaki 2010	8/111	18/98		17.03	0.35 [0.14, 0.83]
Total (95% CI)	632	714		100.00	0.28 [0.16, 0.50]

Total events: 44 (AR group), 160 (NAR group)
Test for heterogeneity: $\chi^2 = 13.53$, df = 7 (p<0.06), $I^2=48.3\%$
Test for overall effect: Z = 4.28 (p<0.0001)

0.1 0.2 0.5 1 2 5 10
Favours AR group   Favours NAR group

Chen J

Study or sub-category	AR n/N	NAR n/N	OR (random) 95% CI	Weight %	OR (random) 95% CI
Kaibori 2006	21/34	112/213		27.12	1.46 [0.69, 3.06]
Regimbeau2002	3/30	17/34		17.45	0.11 [0.03, 0.44]
Tanaka 2008	39/83	25/42		26.95	0.60 [0.28, 1.28]
Wakai 2006	49/95	42/63		28.48	0.53 [0.28, 1.03]
Total (95% CI)	242	352		100.00	0.55 [0.25, 1.23]

Total events: 496 (AR), 363 (NAR)
Test for heterogeneity: Chi² = 16.41, df = 8 (p=0.04), I² = 51.2%
Test for overall effect: Z = 1.50 (p = 0.013)

0.1   0.2   0.5   1   2   5   10

Favours NAR   Favours AR

5.3
Efforts for annihilation of biases in comparison of anatomical and non-anatomical resection

It is thought that there are two major biases present in comparing the oncological outcomes of AR and non-AR. One is on the selection of patients (selection bias), and the other is concerned to the procedural aspect. As the right liver is known to have anatomical variations in numerous cases, compared to the left lobe, surgeons face difficulties in performing ARs quite often. It is surprise that I learned from the literature, that many surgeons are confronted with such concerns as I was.

Ishii et al. compared the prognosis between AR and non-AR. After examining the prognostic factors between two groups, it was confirmed that numerous factors were significantly different between two groups in the first place. An attempt was made to research after eliminating such biases, afterwards. A propensity-score matching (PSM) was used to compare two groups in terms of overall cumulative and disease-free survival. As a result, it was found that there was no statistically significant difference in both cumulative and disease-free survival rates between the two groups (AR and non-AR) in the original study, but after PSM they differed in statistical level (Table 4, Figures 21,22).[11]

Sakai et al., also, attempted to remove the bias. In order to exclude operational (procedure-related) bias due to variation of intrahepatic vasculature in right lobe of the liver, they included HCC patients with tumors in the left lateral section only, comparing the outcome of AR and non-AR. There was no statistically significant difference in the recurrence-free and cumulative survival. However, the cumulative survival showed a near-significant difference with p=0.07. It must be noted that AR was a statistically significant factor in multivariate analysis of factors affecting recurrence rate (Tables 5,6 and Figure 23).[14]

There is no prospective randomized trial in comparing the oncological outcomes of AR and non-AR. However, attempts to reduce biases through multicenter or multinational studies must be continuously undertaken.

Table 4 Clinicopathological characteristics of hepatocellular carcinoma patients who underwent initial hepatectomy in the full analysis set and one-to-one propensity score-matched pairs.[11]

Variables	Full analysis set			Propensity score-matched paris		
	A (n =110)	NA (n = 158)	P value	A (n = 44)	NA (n = 44)	P value
Gender (M:F)	97:13	133:25	0.455	38:6	38:6	NA
Age (yr)	68 (64-70)	66 (64-68)	0.862	64.9 ± 10.2	64.5 ± 9.5	0.838
Etiology (B:C:BC:NBNC)	50:32:1:27	70:61:6:21	0.035	19:18:1:6	24:12:1:7	0.602
Background (N:CH:L)	16:56:38	9:49:100	< 0.001	4:20:20	5:14:25	0.422
Histology (W:M:P)	50:32:27	29:94:35	0.138	6:30:8	8:28:8	0.836
Albumin (mg/ dL)	3.91 ± 0.42	3.86 ± 0.47	0.321	3.99 ± 0.34	3.92 ± 0.41	0.379
Bilirubin (mg/ dL)	0.6 (0.6-0.6)	0.8 (0.7-0.9)	< 0.001	0.68 ± 0.26	0.72 ± 0.39	0.545
PT (%)	93.3 ± 12.2	90.6 ± 13.6	0.106	92.4 ± 11.5	92.5 ± 12.4	0.948
LCGR15 (%)	8.5 (7.4-9.9)	13 (10.8-15)	< 0.001	10.4 ± 5.6	13.5 ± 8.8	0.053
Child-Pugh score (A:B)	109:1	153:5	0.419	44:0	44:0	NA
MELD score	7.68 ± 2.73	7.58 ±1.39	0.674	7.78 ± 3.21	7.37 ± 1.29	0.448
Tumor size (cm)	4.2 (3.5-5.5)	2.5 (2.2-3.0)	< 0.001	3 (2.5-3.5)	3 (2.3-3.5)	0.904
No. of tumors	1 (1-1)	1 (1-1)	0.761	1 (1-1)	1 (1-1)	0.554
VI (-:+:++)	75:18:17	124:25:9	0.027	34:7:3	31:10:3	0.716
OT (min)	400 (364-439)	280 (260-300)	< 0.001	340.1 ± 105.8	322.7 ± 96.8	0.441
Blood loss (mL)	435 (380-600)	300 (230-390)	< 0.001	400 (310-482)	355 (270-560)	0.926
Blood transfusion (U)	1.3 ± 3.6	0.5 ± 2.3	0.049	0.4 ± 1.4	0.5 ± 1.6	0.833
BMI	23.19 ± 3.27	23.61 ± 3.38	0.313	23.57 ± 3.01	22.83 ± 3.13	0.263
Platelets	15.6 (13.3-17.1)	12.6 (11 .7-14.2)	0.504	13.45 ±4.71	16.41 ± 13.69	0.178
AST (IU/ L)	36 (31-41)	36 (31-45)	0.206	40 (33-46)	33 (30-48)	0.439
ALT (IU/ L)	34 (29-38)	32 (28-37)	0.413	38 (32-43)	29 (27-39)	0.103
MELD	7.03 (6.87-7.19)	7.12 (6.87-7.42)	0.674	7.10 (6.87-7.39)	7.03 (6.43-7.29)	0.396
BTR	6.07 (5.60-6.59)	5.42 (5.07-5.84)	< 0.001	5.89 (4.99-6.50)	5.73 (5.06-6.02)	0.277
Hyaluronate (ng/ mL)	98 (76-132)	155 (128-196)	< 0.001	103 (66-139)	137 (104-187)	0.204
HGF (ng/ mL)	0.32 (0.29-0.36)	0.36 (0.32-0.39)	0.069	0.33 ± 0.14	0.39 ± 0.15	0.066
AFP (ng/ mL)	21.2 (11.2-80.9)	13.7 (8-29.5)	0.178	11.7 (6.5-38.4)	14.5 (5.8-46.4)	0.902
PIVKA (mAU/ mL)	228 (90-639)	35 (27-53)	0.015	38 (24-158)	30 (23-66)	0.721

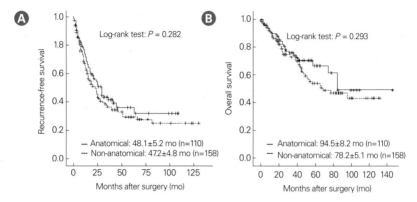

● **Figure 21**   **Recurrence free survival and overall survival in full analysis set in Ishii's paper.**[11]

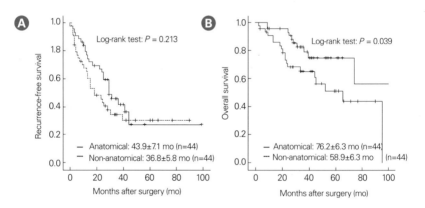

● **Figure 22**   **Recurrence free survival and overall survival in propensity score analysis analysis set in Ishii's paper.**[11]

Table 5 Clinical profiles between anatomical resection and non-anatomical resection in patients with HCC located in the left lateral section.[12]

Variables	Anatomical (n = 30)	Nonanatomical (n = 57)	p
Age	62.0 (36-80)	64.5 (35-80)	0.35
≥ 60/< 60 years	18/12	35/22	1.00
Gender, male/female	18/12	38/19	0.64
HBV infection (positive/negative)	8/22	17/40	0.81
HCV infection (positive/negative)	15/15	29/28	1.00
Child-Pugh classification (A/B)	27/3	42/15	0.10
ICG R15(%) (≥30/<30)	3/27	24/33	<0.01
Platelet counts (µL) (≥105/<105)	23/7	31/26	0.06
AFP (ng/mL) (≥100/<100)	7/23	15/42	0.80
DCP (IU/L) (≥ 100/<100)	7/23	8/45	0.38
Total blood loss (mL)	216 (5-790)	123 (5-942)	<0.01
≥500/<500	4/26	5/52	0.49
Tumor size (cm) ≥3/<3	12/18	11/46	0.05
Tumor differentiation (well or moderate/poor)	19/11	49/8	0.03
Cancer spread (yes/no)	10/20	11/46	0.15
Resection margin width (mm)	5.5 (0-30)	5.0 (0-20)	0.70
≥10 mm/<l0 mm	8/22	20/37	0.48
Liver fibrosis (yes/no)	20/10	54/3	<0.01
Complication (%)	3 (10%)	5 (8.8%)	1.00

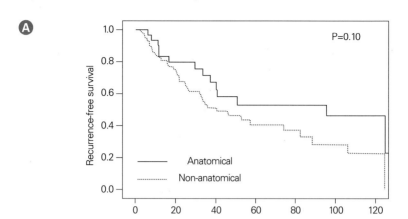

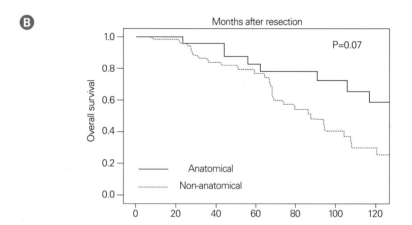

• Figure 23　Comparison of recurrence-free survival (A) and overall survival (B) between anatomical and nonatomical resection for hepatocellular carcinomia limited to the left lateral segment.[12]

Table 6 Univariate and multivariate analysis regardung postoperative prognosis between anatomical resection and nonanatomical resection in patients with HCC located in the left lateral section.[12]

Variables	Patients (no.)	Recurrence				Overall survival			
		Univariate	Multivariate			Univariate	Multivariate		
		P	P	HR	95% CI	P	P	HR	95% CI
Age >60/<60 years	53/34	0.51	0.03	2.08	1.06-4.11	0.51			
Gender, male/female	56/31	0.67				0.23			
HBV infection (yes/no)	19/68	0.89				0.20			
HCV infection (yes/no)	44/43	0.19				0.41			
Child-Pugh classification (A/B)	69/18	0.51				0.03	0.02	2.45	1.16-5.19
ICG R15 [%] (≥30/<30)	27/60	0.57				<0.01			
Platelet counts (µL) (>105/<105)	54/33	0.03				<0.01	0.02	2.23	1.17-4.27
AFP (ng/mL) (≥100/<100)	22/65	0.54				0.35			
DCP (IU/L) (≥100/<100)	15/68	0.71				0.94			
anatomical resection (+/-)	30/57	0.10	0.02	2.36	1.14-4.67	0.07			
Total blood loss (mL) (≥500/<500)	9/78	0.41				0.12			
Tumor size (cm) (≥3/<3)	23/64	0.22				0.98			
Tumor differentiation (well or moderate/poor)	68/19	0.15	0.02	2.54	1.16-4.82	0.68			
Cancer spread (yes/no)	21/66	<0.01	<0.01	2.03	1.38-4.70	<0.01	<0.01	3.45	1.73-6.87
Resection margin width (mm) (≥10/<10)	28/59	0.69				0.34			
Liver fibrosis (yes/no)	74/13	0.15				0.47			
Complication (yes/no)	6/81	0.21				0.88			

5.4
Details of procedure of anatomical resection

Three approaches are used to determine an ideal intersegmental plane during liver resection. First is known as hilar access, ie. Through the hilum. Extrahepatic glissonean sheath is dissected and the portal vein, hepatic artery and bile duct are separated. By clamping the lobar or sectional portal vein the resection plane is identified by ischemic demarcation. This method allow the surgeons to perform hemihepatectomy or sectionectomy. However, access to the hepatic structure beyond the 2nd order branch of portal vein is not possible by this technique. I use this approach mainly for liver resection in hilar cholangiocarcinoma or liver cancer invading the hilum, and also for

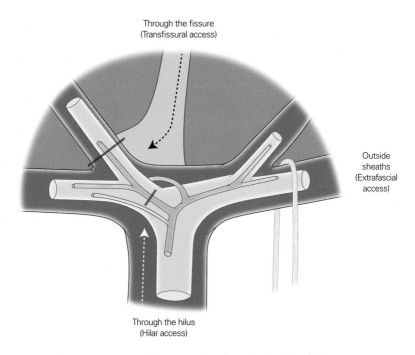

Through the fissure
(Transfissural access)

Outside
sheaths
(Extrafascial
access)

Through the hilus
(Hilar access)

• Figure 24   **Three ways to reach the portal pedicle. (Couinaud C, 1981)**

donor and recipient surgery for liver transplantation. The second method is the extrafascial approach whereby the hilar plate is freed and lowered from the inferior aspect of the liver followed by winding and temporary ligation of 1st, 2nd and 3rd order branches of portal pedicle in sequence and the transection plane is found. While this method is theoretically concise and attractive, it has the burden of dissecting the lower liver parenchyma considerably in the case when the bifurcation of 2nd order branch is furtherly situated during right-side liver surgery; It is not always successful. The third method is the transfissural access: through the fissure. In this method the main portal fissure, right portal fissure and umbilical fissure are to be found by extrafascial approach and they are transsected from the ventral portion of the liver parenchyma. Then, we meet the portal pedicle branches of desired (to be resected) segment(s). By temporary clamping of segmental branches, additional resection plane can be visualized. The second and third methods are referred to as Glissonean approach and are recognized as one of the standard surgical techniques for liver cancer.

To discuss superiority among the different approaches, every technique with a high probability of completing AR despite of variation that might be present can be regarded as a good technique. However, that may depend on each surgeon's preference and familiarity. In my personal experience, I mainly used transfissural approach, while performing extrafascial approach adjunctly. I will discuss the details of the technique in chapter 6.

Anatomical Liver Resection
: Toward Tailored Surgery

6

Personal experience in liver resection

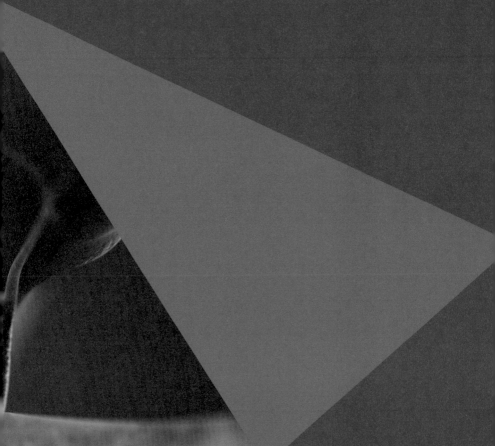

6

Personal experience in liver resection

6.1
Fissural approach of liver resection in early hepatocellular carcinoma

Accoding to Couinaud, a human liver has three fissures (Figure 25): main portal fissure, right portal fissure and umbilical fissure. Transection of the ventral liver parenchyma of the fissures allows a safe access to the target branches of portal pedicle territory of which is to be easily founded. Structurally, the ventral liver is thinner, compared to the dorsal part, and Glissonean pedicles can be easily exposed trough a minor transection of the parenchyma. The main portal fissure is used to perform right and left hemihepatectomy, right anterior sectionectomy, and segmentectomy 5 and 8. Likewise, umbilical fissure is dissected to initiate central bisectionectomy, right trisectionectomy segmentectomy 3, 4, 4 and 5, and left lateral sectionectomy. Lastly, right portal fissure is transected to perform right posterior sectionectomy, left trisectionectomy and segmentectomy 6 and 7 (Figure 25).

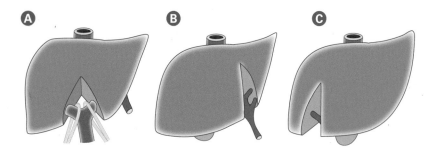

• Figure 25 Glissonean pedicle approach using 3 primary openings of the fissures

(a) Opening of the main portal fissure: Removal of RL, LL, RAS, V and VIII
(b) Opening of the umbilical fissure: Removal of CL, RTS, IV, IV+V, III and LLS
(c) Opening of the right portal fissure: Removal of VI, VII, RPS and LTS

6.2
Modification of procedure according to the anatomical variation

Is AR identical to SR? To answer this question, we need to look back into the anatomical variations of the Glissonean pedicle.

In cases of right and left hemihepatectomy, sectionectomies and monosegmentectomies of the left lobe, AR is identical to SR. Glissonean pedicles to the left lobe have only variations in number of the branches, and discoloration caused by pedicle ligation, always, locates at the plane of left or middle hepatic vein or umbilical fissure. **(Figures 26, 28)**.

As the right liver on the other hand, have a "sliding of origin" type of variations in intrahepatic vasculature, the ischemic demarcation plane is not formed at the right portal fissure or at RHV in about 40% of cases when performing sectionectomies or segmentectomies. In another words, AR is not identical to SR in about 40%. **(Figures 6, 27, 28)**[1]

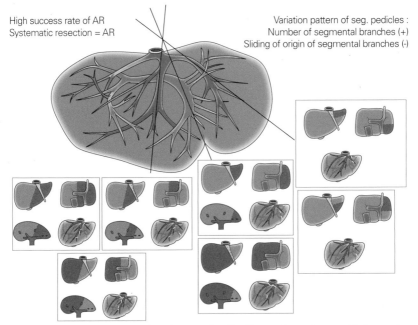

High success rate of AR
Systematic resection = AR

Variation pattern of seg. pedicles :
Number of segmental branches (+)
Sliding of origin of segmental branches (-)

• Figure 26   **Hepatectomies which its resection line lies on the main portal, left portal and umbilical fissures**

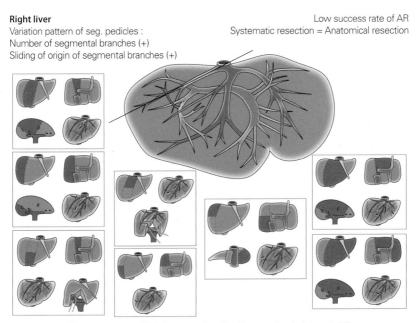

Right liver
Variation pattern of seg. pedicles :
Number of segmental branches (+)
Sliding of origin of segmental branches (+)

Low success rate of AR
Systematic resection = Anatomical resection

• Figure 27   **Hepatectomy which its resection line lies on the right portal fissure**

Let's take right anterior sectionectomy (RAS), for example to take a look at the anatomical variation of the right lobe and contemplate the way to overcome. The upper diagram of the **figure 29** shows a typical vascular structure of a liver. In this example, AR and SR are identical procedures. The lower diagram shows a hypertrophied right anterior portal pedicle which crosses the border into the RPS. In such case, SR of RAS exceeds AR. However, the RHV can easily be exposed at the resection

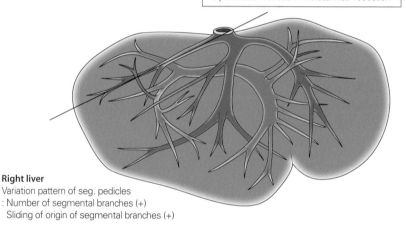

Left liver
Variation pattern of seg. pedicles
: Number of segmental branches (+)
  Sliding of origin of segmental branches (-)

High success rate of AR
Systematic resection = Anatomical resection

Right liver
Variation pattern of seg. pedicles
: Number of segmental branches (+)
  Sliding of origin of segmental branches (+)

Low success rate of AR
Systematic resection ≠ Anatomical resection

• Figure 28   **Anatomical variation of intrahepatic Glisson pedicles**

When resection line of hepatectomy lies on the right portal fissure, it is difficult for us to do AR in about 40% cases. Therefore, the success rate of AR is somewhat low.

margin (Figure 29). Conversely, if the right posterior portal pedicle is hypertrophied, a SR of RAS becomes smaller than AR. RHV cannot be exposed in the field, when performing RAS in this case. Therefore, AR and SR of RAS in RPS-hypertrophied liver are not identical, and it is SR but not AR, strictly speaking. However, if the violation is not large, we regard it as an AR. (near-anatomical resection)

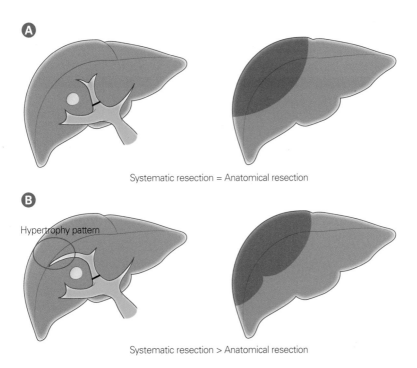

Systematic resection = Anatomical resection

Systematic resection > Anatomical resection

• Figure 29   **Hypertrophied segmental pedicle**

Next, I would like to discuss the "sliding of origin" pattern of variation in the right lobe of the liver. The upper diagram of **figure 30** shows a small RPS branch arising from right anterior portal pedicle. In this case, ligation of right anterior portal pedicle may cause an extensive discoloration of the right lobe. If a surgeon intends to perform a SR of RAS, sparing the RHV, an excess of liver parenchyma anterior to the RHV can be resected: This type of operation can hardly be regarded as an AR nor SR. De-vascularized liver tissue anterior to the RHV can be left which violates the definition of an SR. Meanwhile, the resected territory exceeds the anatomical RAS territory making it difficult to meet the rule of an AR. In case of right anterior sectionectomy in the liver with a "sliding RAS branch to RPS", I suggest classify it as a non-AR.

I prefer to initiate the liver resection (RAS) by transecting the main portal

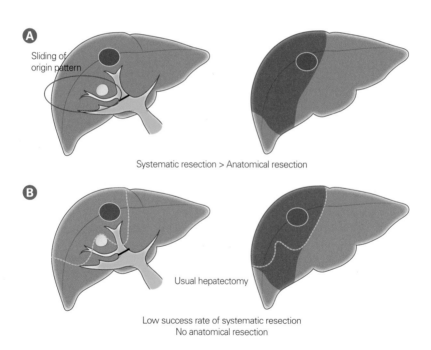

A

Sliding of origin pattern

Systematic resection > Anatomical resection

B

Usual hepatectomy

Low success rate of systematic resection
No anatomical resection

• Figure 30 **Posterior segmental pedicle slidden to anterior portal pedicle (anterior dominant pattern)**

fissure in this case with above mentioned "sliding of origin" pattern of variation (**Figure 31**). As the transection is continued, along the anterior aspect of anterior branch of glissonean pedicle is exposed. Then, the transection plane is tilted and continued to the depth of 1 to 2 centimeters to right side, exposing the right anterior portal pedicle. At this point the sliding RPS branch can be met. By ligating the right anterior portal pedicle just distal of the origin of the slidden branch, an SR and AR can be done without additional parenchyma damage. An example of the operation field is shown in **figure 32. Figure 33** shows the process of right anterior portal pedicle ligation preserving the sliding branch after transfissural approach. Couinaud, also, mentioned this technique and named it an "open-book method".

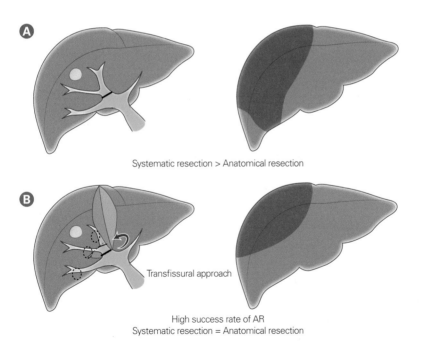

Systematic resection > Anatomical resection

Transfissural approach

High success rate of AR
Systematic resection = Anatomical resection

• Figure 31 **Transfissural approach to overcome anatomical variations of sliding of origin (anterior dominant type)**

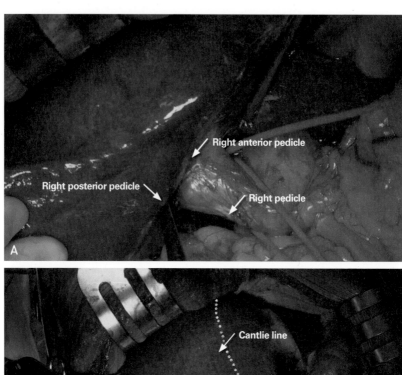

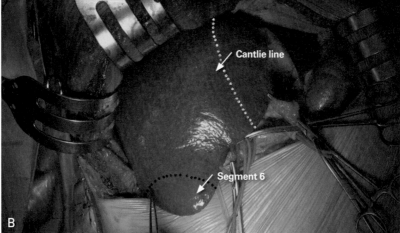

• **Figure 32-1 Transfissural approach to overcome anatomical variations of sliding of origin**

A. Hilar dissection and Looping anterior and posterior pedicles, respectively. B. Discolored anterior surface of the liver: discoloration of near-entire liver surface except small part of segment 6. C. Counter-staining of the posterior pedicle. D. Discolored small part of segment 6.

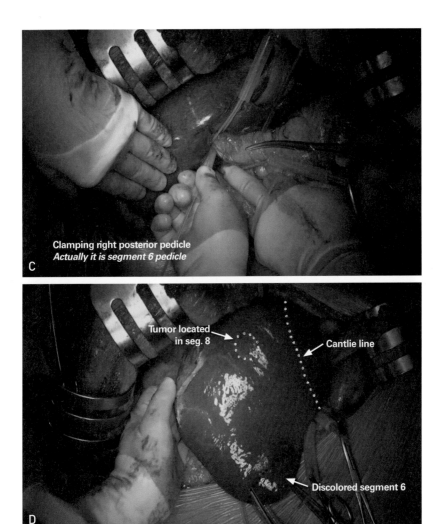

C — Clamping right posterior pedicle
Actually it is segment 6 pedicle

D — Tumor located in seg. 8 — Cantlie line — Discolored segment 6

• **Figure 32-1** **Transfissural approach to overcome anatomical variations of sliding of origin**

A. Hilar dissection and Looping anterior and posterior pedicles, respectively. B. Discolored anterior surface of the liver: discoloration of near-entire liver surface except small part of segment 6. C. Counter-staining of the posterior pedicle. D. Discolored small part of segment 6.

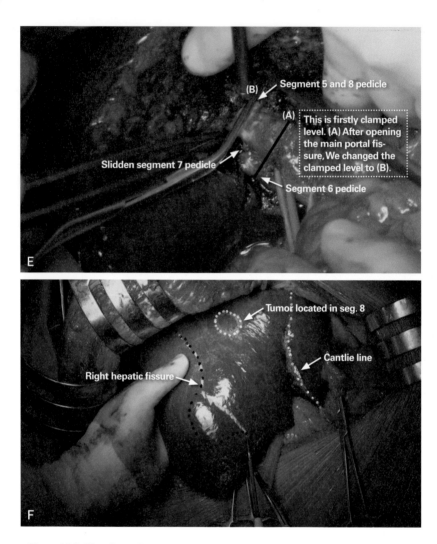

Figure 32-2 Transfissural approach to overcome anatomical variations of sliding of origin

E. Through opening the main portal fissure and exposing the anterior pedicle, we identified slidden branch of the posterior pedicle, and clamped the anterior pedicle just distal of the origin of the slidden pedicle. F. Newly discolored surface of the anterior segment. G. operative field after anterior sectionectomy.

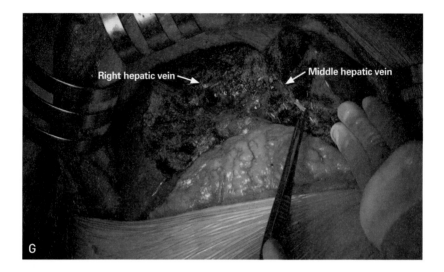

• **Figure 32-2 Transfissural approach to overcome anatomical variations of sliding of origin**
E. Through opening the main portal fissure and exposing the anterior pedicle, we identified slidden branch of the posterior pedicle, and clamped the anterior pedicle just distal of the origin of the
slidden pedicle. F. Newly discolored surface of the anterior segment. G. operative field after anterior
sectionectomy.

There are cases where a branch or branches of RAS originate(s) from the
right posterior portal pedicle. In such cases, clamping of the right anterior
portal pedicle results in partial discoloration of anatomical RAS. If the tumor is
confined to the discolored territory, resection of the territory is an acceptable
choice. It is an SR, but not an AR. If the tumor is not confined or the surgeon
intends to perform an AR, an artificial plane containing the RHV can be used
to complete right anterior sectionectomy as shown in the lower diagram of
Figure 34. Strictly speaking, this cannot be classified as an AR nor SR.

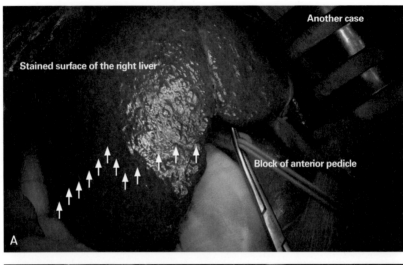

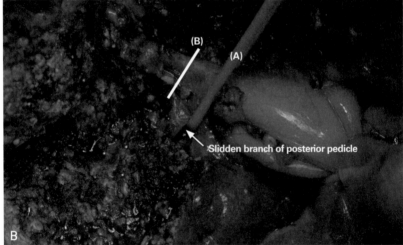

After hepatotomy through the portal fissure, we can open the liver like a book. (Couinaud C)

• **Figure 33 Preservation of slidden posterior pedicle through transfissural approach (another case)**

A. After block of anterior pedicle, discoloration of near-entire surface of the right liver except small part of posterior section. B. (a) Firstly clamped level in the extrafascial approach. After opening the main portal fissure, we changed the clamped level to (b).

To overcome this difficulty, I use transfissural approach. The main portal fissure is dissected to expose the anterior surface of the right Glissonean pedicle. The transection line is switched to the right side. Further dissection exposes the right anterior pedicle. After its ligation and division, the parenchymal transection is continued exposing the right posterior pedicle. The slidden variant branch can be visualized at this point. Ligation of slidden branch

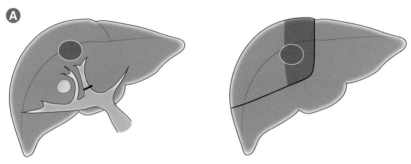

Systematic resection < Anatomical resection

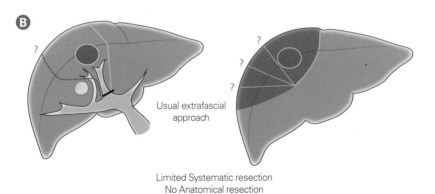

Usual extrafascial approach

Limited Systematic resection
No Anatomical resection

• **Figure 34   Anterior segmental pedicle slidden to posterior portal pedicle (posterior dominant pattern)**

It is difficult for us to make the anatomical right margin using conventional approach.

completes the AR. An example of the procedure is shown in **Figure 36**.

Modification in procedures as mentioned above allows the surgeons to overcome the "sliding of origin" pattern of varation in many ways. In my opinion, compromized procedures must be classified as non-ARs.

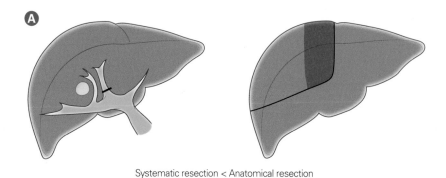

Systematic resection < Anatomical resection

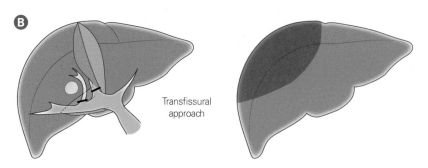

High success rate of AR
Systematic resection = Anatomical resection

• Figure 35 **Transfissural approach to overcome anatomical variations of sliding of origin (Posterior dominant type)**

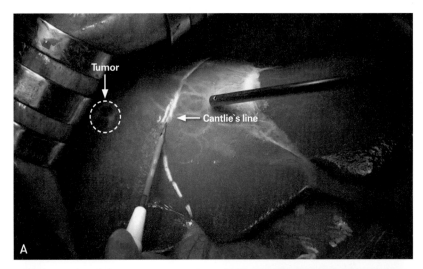

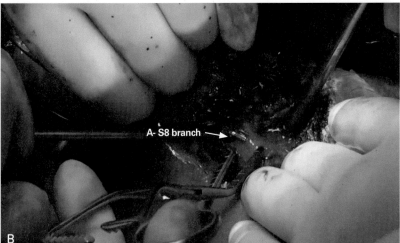

• **Figure 36-1 Transfissural approach to overcome anatomical variations of sliding of origin (posterior dominant type)**

A. After hilar dissection and clamping the right pedicle, discolored right liver. B. After dissection of dorsal part of the Cantlie line for segmentectomy 8 using Takasaki's approach, identified segment 8 portal pedicle. C. In spite of clamping of segment 8 pedicle, the only small part of segment 8 was discolored. D. After decision of anterior sectionectomy, we clamped anterior pedicle. But, the only small part of anterior section was discolored.

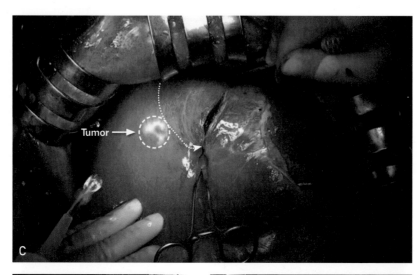

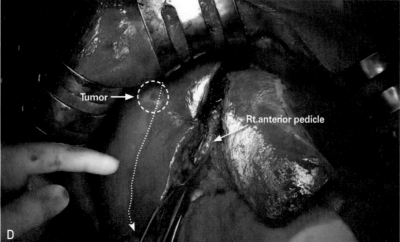

- **Figure 36-1   Transfissural approach to overcome anatomical variations of sliding of origin (posterior dominant type)**

A. After hilar dissection and clamping the right pedicle, discolored right liver. B. After dissection of dorsal part of the Cantlie line for segmentectomy 8 using Takasaki's approach, identified segment 8 portal pedicle. C. In spite of clamping of segment 8 pedicle, the only small part of segment 8 was discolored. D. After decision of anterior sectionectomy, we clamped anterior pedicle. But, the only small part of anterior section was discolored.

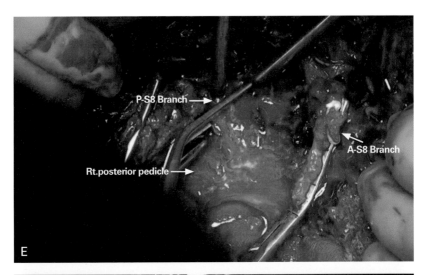

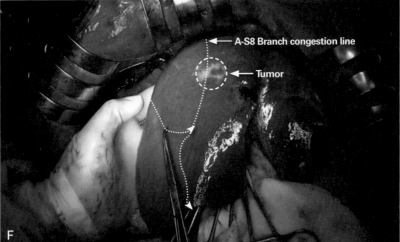

• Figure 36-2 **Transfissural approach to overcome anatomical variations of sliding of origin (posterior dominant type)**

E. After dicision of anterior pedicle, we dissected to right side exposing the anterosuperior surface of the posterior sectional pedicle. After 1.5cm dissection, we can identified slidden anterior portal pedicle. It was clamped, F. After additional clamping of the slidden branch, the changed discolored liver surface was shown. G. The operative field after anterior sectionectomy.

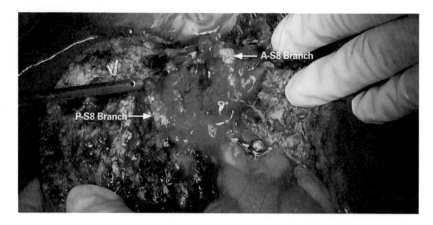

• **Figure 36-2 Transfissural approach to overcome anatomical variations of sliding of origin (posterior dominant type)**

E. After dicision of anterior pedicle, we dissected to right side exposing the anterosuperior surface of the posterior sectional pedicle. After 1.5cm dissection, we can identified slidden anterior portal pedicle. It was clamped, F. After additional clamping of the slidden branch, the changed discolored liver surface was shown. G. The operative field after anterior sectionectomy.

6.3
Outcomes of surgical treatment of hepatocellular carcinoma

854 liver resections for HCC were performed in my institution in the duration of 19 years from July 1995 to July 2014. The male to female ratio was 3.74 to 1. The mean age of patients was 52, and 72% of them had chronic hepatitis B. 64.8% had liver cirrhosis. Operative mortality was 1.05%. AJCC staging distribution was 33.4% in stage 1, 35.6% in stage 2, 19.0% in stage 3 and 12.0% in stage 4, respectively **(Table 7)**.

Subjects with single HCC, less than 5cm were selected to compare the outcomes of AR and non-AR. This measure was taken to reduce bias by the stage of HCC. Finally 397 patients were enrolled in the study. AR was performed in 247 cases (62.4%) and non-AR was performed in 150 (37.6%). Reasons for performing non-AR were mostly due to compromised

Table 7　Clinical profiles of HCC patients with patial hepatectomy

Personal experience: 854 cases	
Male:Female	674:180 (3.74:1)
Age	mean 52 years
Etiology B-viral	636 cases (74.5%)
C-viral	51 cases (6.0%)
B- & C-viral	4 cases (0.5%)
Non-viral	171 cases (20.0%)
Cirrhosis(+)	553 cases (64.8%)
AFP > 20 ng/ml	478 cases (56.0%)
Hospital mortality	9 cases (1.05%)
AJCC staging I:II:III:IV	285:304:162:103 (33.4%:35.6%:19.0%:12.0%)

* *These data were collected consecutively and prospectively in Ajou University Hospital.*

(Ajou University Hospital: July 1995 – July 2014)

Table 8　Outcomes after hepatectomy in Ajou University Hospital

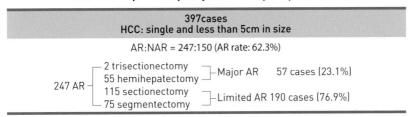

397cases
HCC: single and less than 5cm in size

AR:NAR = 247:150 (AR rate: 62.3%)

247 AR
- 2 trisectionectomy
- 55 hemihepatectomy — Major AR　57 cases (23.1%)
- 115 sectionectomy
- 75 segmentectomy — Limited AR 190 cases (76.9%)

(Ajou University Hospital: July 1995 – July 2014)

liver function. Some of the non-AR groups had variations in intrahepatic vasculature, impossible to overcome (Table 8). I mainly used transfissural approach to ensure high success rate of AR. In most of the cases, extrafascial access was used in conjunction in order to find the fissures. A strict criterion of AR was applied in all cases (Figure 24, 25).

A PSM was applied to reduce biases in comparing the outcomes of AR and non-AR (Table 9). In the analysis of total patients, AR was superior to the non-AR in terms of disease-free survival. However, no statistically significant difference was found in cumulative survival rate **(Figure 37)**. After PSM, the outcome of AR was more favorable in both disease-free and cumulative survival. **(Figure 38)**.

Table 9   Clinicopathological characteristics of single and less than 5cm HCC patients who underwent hepatectomy in the full analysis set and one-to-one propensity score matched pairs.

	Baseline characteristics (Total patients/non-matching)			Baseline characteristics (PS matching)		
	AR	NAR	p_value	AR	NAR	p_value
Patients (no.)	247	150	0	200	200	1
(%)	62.22	37.78-		50	50-	
Age (mean)	52.36	53.6	0.213	52.05	52.84	0.442
(sd)	9.52	9.69-		10.18	10.36-	
Sex	180	127	0.002	145	172	0.129
(%)	58.63	41.37-		45.74	54.26-	
LLS_Location	36	19	0.022	31	30	0.898
(%)	65.45	34.55-		50.82	49.18-	
recur	93	72	0.102	83	107	0.082
(%)	56.36	43.64-		43.68	56.32-	
death	67	35	0.002	36	58	0.023
(%)	65.69	34.31-		38.3	61.7	
Tumorsize (mean)	2.97	2.76	0.07	3.08	3.1	0.88
(sd)	1.14	1.07-		1.08	1.1-	
Albumin (mean)	2.97	2.76	0.07	3.08	3.1	0.88
(sd)	0.63	0.5-	0.46	0.4-		
Bilirubin (mean)	1.46	0.92	0.018	0.81	0.81	0.986
(sd)	3.51	0.6-		0.64	0.49-	
PT (mean)	13.3	12.72	0.022	12.47	12.43	0.762
(sd)	3.31	1.63-		1.51	1.35-	
Platelet (mean)	127129.3	140133.3	0.07	149022.1	144495	0.442
(sd)	81522.52	60385.53-		68122.42	47719.45-	
AST (mean)	51	48.81	0.56	47.97	45.16	0.444
(sd)	42.11	32.05-		42.98	29.02-	
ALT (mean)	49.05	50.99	0.615	50.15	47.37	0.463
(sd)	40.38	35.08-		42.92	32.12-	
AFP (mean)	1010.64	768.3	0.552	1203.96	777.08	0.256
(sd)	3327.59	4262.02-		3665.77	3844.57-	
Rupture	6	5	0.763			
(%)	54.55	45.45-				

(Ajou University Hospital: 1995-2012)

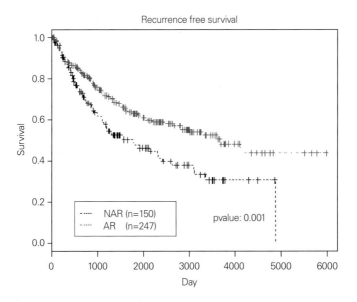

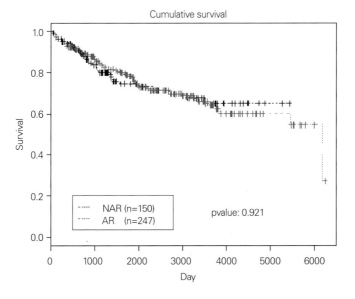

• Figure 37 **Recurrence free survival and overall survival in full analysis set**

(Ajou University Hospital: 1995-2012)

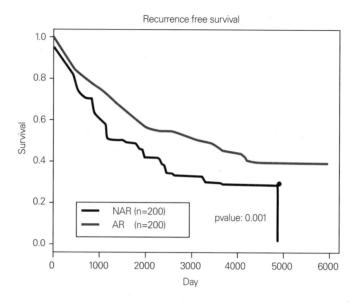

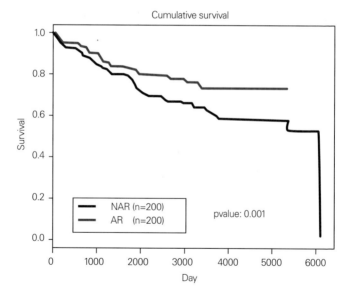

• Figure 38   **Recurrence free survival and overall survival in propensity score analysis analysis set**

(Ajou University Hospital: 1995-2012)

6.4
Conclusion

I believe that the AR or SR is critical to ensure a better oncological outcome. I had put effort in raising the success rate of AR despite the anatomical variation whenever liver function is acceptable. Glissonean approach through transfissural access and PSM analysis are useful in overcoming selection and operative biases. Moreover, a positive oncological effect of AR can be revealed by applying a strict criterion for AR.

Anatomical Liver Resection
: Toward Tailored Surgery

7

Videos of liver resection
by fissural/Glissonean approaches

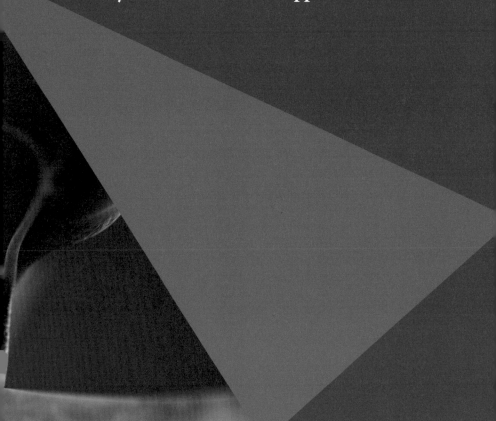

7

Videos of liver resection by fissural/Glissonean approaches

Details of patient management before and after liver resection are omitted in this book. Instead, technical aspect of liver resection is dealt. A hockey-stick incision is preferred. A midline incision extending from the xyphoid process to the half way down to umbilicus, combined with a subcostal incision is optimal in exposing the operative field. During laparotomy, the umbilical ligament is ligated and dissected from the anterior surface of the liver for retraction. Three arms of Kent retractor are installed at 2, 10 and 11 o'clock direction. Right or left coronary and triangular ligaments are taken down and the roots of hepatic veins; right, middle and left are dissected and exposed. Intraoperative ultrasound is used to identify the location of the tumor and possible vascular invasion or thrombosis. Pringle maneuver is used only if excessive hemorrhage is expected or seen during parenchymal transection. Parenchymal division is performed using CUSA in both open and laparoscopic (or robotic) surgery. Occasionally water-jet dissector is used. Crushing technique using a Kelly clamp is preferred when exposing the hepatic veins and their tributaries. After extraction of specimen, resection margin hemostasis follows. Argon beam laser and bipolar coagulator are useful for bleeding control. Afterwards, fibrin glue is sprayed and 2 silastic Jackson-Pratt drains are inserted. Details of surgery and videos are shown below.

7.1
Right hemihepatectomy (Figure 39)

This is a case of a huge HCC that is located adjacent to the diaphragm and stretching inferiorly to the liver hilum. Therefore, an anterior approach without right lobe mobilization is adopted. After cholecystectomy, right portal pedicle (1st order branch) is temporarily clamped to find the Cantlie's line. Parenchymal transection is initiated at the anterior surface following the ischemic demarcation line. Retraction of the round ligament to the left side is helpful in making a fair operative field. When the parenchymal

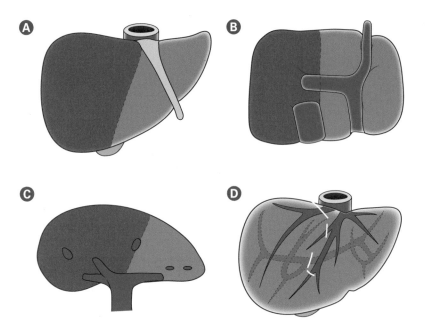

• Figure 39   **Right hepatectomy (Couinaud C, 1981)**

a and b. Territory to be resected seen on the superior and inferior surfaces of the liver.
c. Territoy to be resected seen in a frontal section through the hilum.
d. The vessels to be divided.

dissection meets Glissonean sheath at its superior aspect, dissection plane is tilted to right side, exposing right anterior portal pedicle. Right anterior portal pedicle is then clamped and ligated at the root. The resected pedicle is repaired with 5-0 prolene continuous suture. Parenchymal dissection is continued exposing the right posterior portal pedicle, and it's ligated in the same way. It is highly recommended that right anterior and posterior pedicles are ligated separately instead of ligating at the common right pedicle trunk owing to possible variation in hepatic artery, portal vein and bile duct within the 1st order branch of Glisson's sheath. Further division of liver parenchyma reaches inferior vena cava (IVC). At this point, hanging maneuver is applied, and parenchymal transection is continued to the caudal direction until the IVC is exposed in whole length. RHV is divided between vascular clamps, and the right lobe is freed. After extraction of the specimen, the cut edge of RHV is repaired with a 5-0 prolene continuous suture.

7.2
Left hemihepatectomy (Figure 40)

After cholecystectomy, hilar Glissonean pedicles are freed from the hilar plate, and the left portal pedicle is encircled with nelaton catheter. Temporary clamping of the left portal pedicle visualizes the main portal fissure. Relation between the main portal fissure and the MHV is confirmed by ultrasound. Ventral dissection of the main portal fissure allows access to the suprahilar Glissonean pedicle. The parenchymal transection plane is tilted to the left side, perpendicularly, and the paracaval portion of the caudate lobe is preserved making a plane parallel to the anterior line of hilum and the Arantius duct. It is critical to spare the MHV. Operator's right index finger is inserted encircling the left portal pedicle confirming the Arantius duct. In this level, left portal pedicle is divided, overcoming the variation within the Glissonean sheath. The stump of left portal pedicle is closed by a continuous suture with 5-0 prolene. Further transection along the Arnatius duct, retracting the left lobe to the left

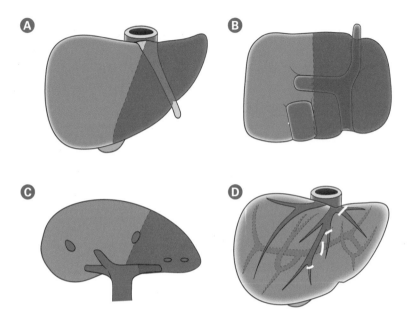

• Figure 40   **Left hepatectomy (Couinaud C, 1981)**

a and b. Territory to be resected seen on the superior and inferior surfaces of the liver;
the caudate lobe which may be removed or retained is darker.
c. Territoy to be resected seen in a frontal section through the hilum.
d. The vessels to be divided.

side exposes the root of LHV. Careful division of LHV is needed in order not to disrupt the MHV. After extraction of the left lobe, LHV stump is repaired with 5-0 prolene continuous suture.

7.3
Central bisectionectomy (Figure 41)

Hilar Glissonean pedicle is encircled with a nelaton tube, and cholecystectomy is performed. The liver parenchyma is, then, dissected along the right side of round ligament, and Glissonean branches of

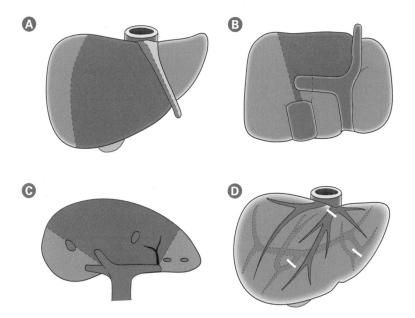

• Figure 41   **Central bisectionectomy (Couinaud C, 1981)**

a and b. Territory to be resected seen on the superior and inferior surfaces of the liver.
Transection on the left is through the umbilical fissure, and that on the right through the right portal fissure.
c. Territoy to be resected seen in a frontal section through the hilum.
d. The vessels to be divided.

segment 4 are ligated and divided using manual ties or vascular clips. Parenchyma is transected until suprahilar Glissonean sheath is exposed, and the transection plane is tilted to the right side to reach the right anterior pedicle. Right anterior pedicle is clamped and divided and stump is repaired with 5-0 prolene continuous suture. Sparing of RHV is crucial. Ultrasound allows localization of the RHV. Bleeding from the resection margin can be controlled by electrocauterization. The specimen containing the right anterior section and segment 4 can be extracted after completion of parenchyma division upto the anterior surface of the confluence portion between RHV and retrohepatic IVC.

7.4
Right anterior sectionectomy (Figure 42)

The right liver is mobilized and cholecystectomy is performed. Hilar Glissonean pedicle is encircled with a nelaton catheter. Right Glissonean pedicle is temporarily clamped to find the main portal fissure. Intraoperative ultrasound is performed to observe the MHV and its relation with the main portal fissure. Ventral parenchyma of the main portal fissure is transected, preserving the MHV. In the video, the patient's right anterior pedicle is a wide fan-like shape rather than a chord-like structure, and there are multiple Glissonean branches of segment 8. Although it is difficult to perform the procedure, the anterior pedicle

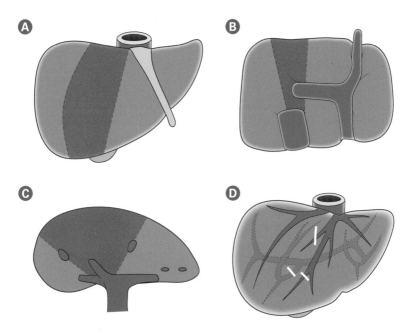

• Figure 42   **Right anterior sectionectomy (Couinaud C, 1981)**

a and b. Territory to be resected seen on the superior and inferior surfaces of the liver.
c. Territoy to be resected seen in a frontal section through the hilum.
d. The vessels to be divided.

is divided without problems. The stump was repaired with 5-0 prolene suture. Afterwards, discolored RAS is seen with the right portal fissure to the right side. Right portal fissure was transsected sparing the RHV until the IVC is exposed at the superior aspect of the liver. RAS is, then, extracted.

7.5
Right posterior sectionectomy (Figure 43)

A Hockey-stick incision is made, and the right liver is mobilized. Cholecystectomy is performed. The hilar plate is lowered. The right posterior

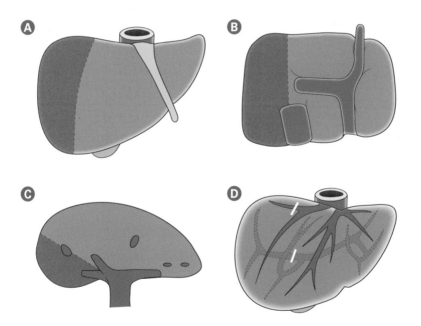

• Figure 43   **Right posterior sectionectomy (Couinaud C, 1981)**

a and b. Territory to be resected seen on the superior and inferior surfaces of the liver.
c.Territoy to be resected seen in a frontal section through the hilum.
d. The vessels to be divided.

pedicle is encircled with a nelaton catheter. Temporary clamping of the right posterior pedicle discolors the RPS, visualizing the right portal fissure. Ultrasound is done in order to observe the tumor and its relation to RHV. The 1st order branch of the right pedicle is strangled to reduce the hemorrhage (Right hemi-block), and right portal fissure is transected. When the right posterior portal pedicle is exposed, it is divided between the clamps and suture ligated. Transection of parenchyma continues until the RHV is exposed and right posterior section is, then, extracted.

7.6
Segmentectomy 1 (Figure 44)

Segmentectomy 1 does not require fissural approach. After laparotomy, liver is mobilized. Cholecystectomy follows, and the hilar main pedicle is encircled with a nelaton catheter. Hilar glissonean pedicle is detached from the hilar plate. Temporary clamping of the right posterior pedicle allows counter-staining (ischemic demarcation) of the right posterior section, visualizing the border between the right posterior section and caudate lobe. The demarcation plane is the transection plane. Intraoperative ultrasound is helpful in identifying the relation between the transection plane and the RHV. The surrounding soft tissue and short hepatic veins of the Spiegel lobe are ligated and divided, and lesser sac is dissected to ligate the Arantius ligament in the just anterior to the IVC. Right liver is, then, pulled anteriorly and three black silk 4-0 sutures are stayed near the resection line of the paracaval portion of the caudate lobe for retraction. Parenchymal transection is performed along the demarcated plane. During the transection, the posterior surface of RHV may be exposed, preserving it, and the caudate branches of the glissonean are ligated and divided. In the past, I use to perform caudate lobectomy by following a parallel plane to the Arantius ligament from the left side of the liver or by starting parenchymal transection from inferior to superior direction which is known as the Gulch approach. However, after T. Takayama's literature, I prefer to use the approach as

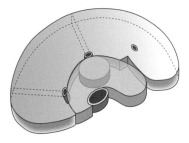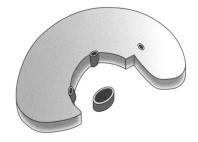

• **Figure 44   Isolated caudate lobectomy (Takayama T, 1981)**

a. In this schema, the tumor is identified at the paracaval portion of the caudate lobe.adjacent to the middle hepatic vein.
b. After transection of the caudate lobe, the dorsal sides of the middle and right hepatic veins are exposed,
and both major lobes and completely separated from from the inferior vena cava.

above mentioned. The advantage of this approach is that it allows a fair view of the hepatic veins making it easier to prevent injuries.

7.7
Segmentectomy 2 (Figure 45)

After laparotomy, the ligaments of left lobe of the liver are dissected to mobilize the liver. The round ligament is dissected and clamped for retraction. It is pulled to the right anterior direction and parenchymal transection is performed caudo-cranially at the left side of the umbilical fissure, using a waterjet dissector. When the portal pedicle to the segment 3 (P3) is exposed at the operative field, it is temporarily clamped for counter-staining of the segment 2. The dissection plane between the segments 2 and 3 is seen. Intraoperative ultrasound is useful in identifying the relation between this transection plane and the LHV. Parenchymal transection is commenced from the ventral portion exposing the posterior surface of the LHV. The LHV tributaries from the segment 2 are carefully ligated and divided, preserving the

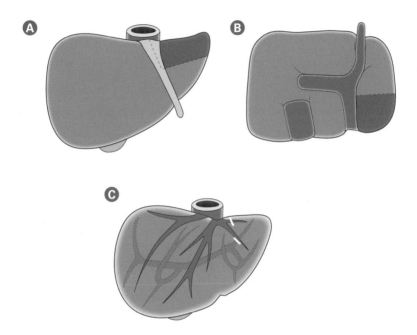

• Figure 45　Segmentectomy 2 (Couinaud C. 1981)

a and b. Territory to be resected seen on the superior and inferior surfaces of the liver.
c. The vessels to be divided.

LHV. The segment 2 Glisson pedicles are divided and ligated in their roots. Transection is complete by exposing the confluence of LHV trunk and IVC.

7.8
Segmentectomy 4 (Figure 46)

After laparotomy, intraoperative ultrasound is performed in order to identify the location of the tumor and its relation to the MHV. Cholecystectomy follows, and parenchymal transection is started from the right border of the umbilical fissure. Encountered Glissonean pedicle branches to the segment

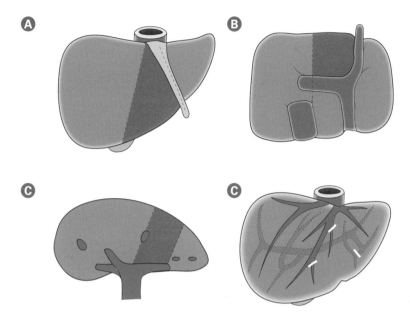

Figure 46   **Left medial sectionectomy (Segmentectomy 4) (Couinaud C. 1981)**

a and b. Territory to be resected seen on the superior and inferior surfaces of the liver.
c. Territoy to be resected seen in a frontal section through the hilum.
d. The vessels to be divided.

4 (P4s) are ligated and divided in the order of appearance with silk ties or vascular clips. The transection plane is switched perpendicularly to right side after encountering the suprahilar Glissonean sheath. This makes the ventral border of the caudate lobe which is parallel to the Arantius ligament and the hilum. The transection continues to the root of the right anterior portal pedicle. Dissection of the main portal fissure is performed afterwards. The main portal fissure at this point is visible due to the ischemic demarcation of the segment 4. The MHV can be exposed at the dissection plane. All segment 4 tributaries are to be ligated and divided. Completion of the main portal fissure transection allows specimen extraction.

7.9
Segmentectomy 5 (Figure 47)

After laparotomy, intraoperative ultrasound is performed in order to identify the location of the tumor. Cholecystectomy follows, and the hilum is lowered to encircle the right Glissonean pedicle with a nelaton catheter. The right

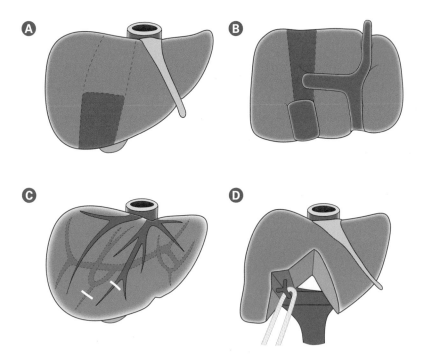

• **Figure 47   Segmentectomy 5 (Couinaud C. 1981)**

a and b. Territory to be resected seen on the superior and inferior surfaces of the liver.
c. The vessels to be divided.
d. Following opening the main portal fissure, passage of a the nelaton tube around the anterior Glisson pedicle; a lateral slit
exposes the anterior surface of the sheath in order to reach the anterior branches, especially segment 5 pedicles.

anterior pedicle is separated and temporarily clamped. The ischemic change of the RAS visualizes the main and right portal fissure which are the left and right border of the segment 5. Transection is started at the ventral portion of the main portal fissure. By exposing the right anterior pedicle, all branches to segment 5 are ligated. In the process, the ischemic demarcation of the segment 5 is seen, visualizing the transverse plane of the caudal border of the segment 5. The transverse transection, then, follows up to the right portal fissure mobilizing the segment 5. Thereafter, the right portal fissure is opened caudo-cranially, allowing segment 5 extraction.

7.10
Segmentectomy 6 (Figure 48)

After laparotomy, cholecystectomy is done. Right lobe of the liver is sufficiently mobilized. Intraoperative ultrasound is used to identify the location of the tumor and its relation to surrounding vascular structure. Right posterior portal pedicle can be temporarily clamped using extrafascial approach in search of the right portal fissure. Sometimes, a branch of right posterior pedicle can be seen at the Rouviere groove. Clamping of this branch discolors a part of the RPS. Either way can visualize the right portal fissure. After finding the fissure, it is dissected from the ventral portion, until the right posterior portal pedicle is exposed. Its branches to segment 6 (P6s) are ligated and divided in order of appearance, and the border between the segments 6 and 7 can be identified. Transection of this border allows extraction of the segment 6.

Two videos are shown that uses clamping of the right posterior pedicle and an approach through Rouviere groove, respectively (segmentectomy 6: part 1 and 2).

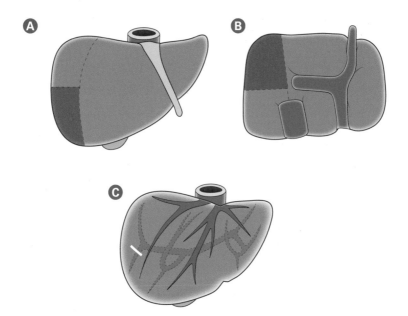

• **Figure 48** **Segmentectomy 6 (Couinaud C. 1981)**

a and b. Territory to be resected seen on the superior and inferior surfaces of the liver.
As the right portal fissure is oblique, this segment extends more in the inferior surface than in the superior surface.
c. The vessels to be divided.

7.11
Segmentectomy 7 (Figure 49, 51)

Anatomical resection of the segment 7 is the least successful procedure of all segmentectomies, although definition of the anatomical resection may vary. Two approaches are used in our institution. The first approach is Takasaki's approach. Glisson sheath is lowered from the hilar plate and the right posterior pedicle is separated. Temporary clamping of the right posterior pedicle induces ischemic demarcation of the RPS showing the right portal fissure. The superior aspect of the right portal fissure is dissected and the surgeon finds the P7. Ligation and division of P7 follows and further dissection

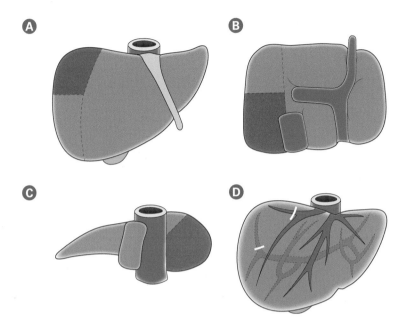

• **Figure 49 Segmentectomy 7 (Couinaud C. 1981)**

a and b. Territory to be resected seen on the superior and inferior surfaces of the liver.
c. Territoy to be resected seen on the posterior surface of the liver.
d. The vessels to be divided.

along the discolored plane exposing the right surface of the RHV completes segmentectomy 7 (Figure 6). Second approach is ultrasound-guided method. It is used when finding P7 by above mentioned approach is unpliant or in case of severe liver fibrosis. Ultrasound probe is applied to 1/2 area of right portal fissure in search of the bifurcation point of P6 and P7. Parenchymal transection is performed along the plane perpendicular to the right portal fissure. After ligation and division of P7, the dissection line follows RHV. After completion of the segmentectomy 7, the dissection plane is coagulated with an argon-beam laser or a bipolar coagulator. Tachocomb seal or fibrin glue can be applied afterwards.

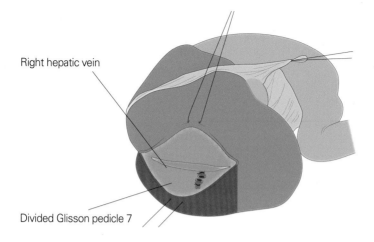

Right hepatic vein

Divided Glisson pedicle 7

● Figure 50　**Segmentectomy 7 using Takasaki approach**

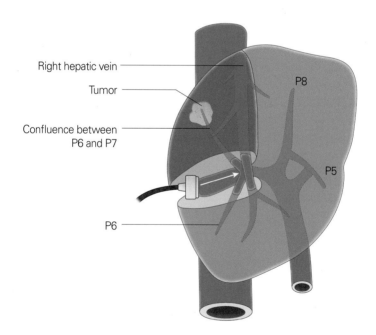

Right hepatic vein

Tumor

Confluence between
P6 and P7

P6

P8

P5

● Figure 51　**Segmentectomy 7 using intraoperative ultrasound**

7.12
Segmentectomy 8 (Figure 52, 53)

In order to apply an extrafascial approach of the segmentectomy 8, an extensive parenchymal division is needed to expose the segmental Glissonean pedicle (P8). This may result in an excessive amount of bleeding which is difficult to halt. Even so, the success rate of AR is low. Professor Takasaki mentioned in his writing about a technique whereby the main portal fissure is detected through clamping right portal pedicle to induce ischemic demarcation of the right lobe. After dissection of the superior-ventral half of the main portal fissure, the root of P8 is found, ligated and divided which resulted in the discoloration of right and anterior border of the segment 8. On the other hand, Professor Makuuchi uses indocyanine green (ICG) dye

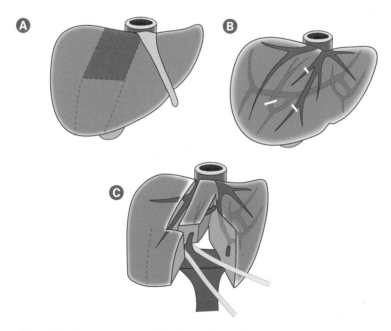

• **Figure 52   Segmentectomy 8 (Couinaud C. 1981)**

a. Territory to be resected.
b. The vessels to be divided.
c. Opening the fissures and detachment of the segment 8.

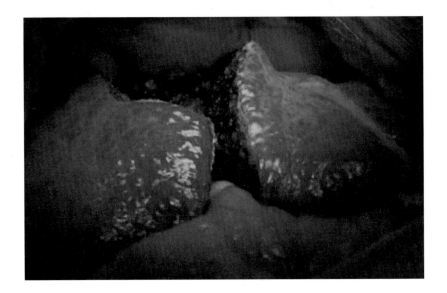

• **Figure 53   Segmentectomy 8**

The postoperative field after segment 8 using transfissural technique.

injection technique. Under intraoperative ultrasound, ICG is injected to the P8 which discolors the segment 8, and parenchymal transection is performed along the border of discolored liver surface until P8 root is found. In my experience without 3D images, both method are somewhat difficult to use and the success rate was not high. Therefore, I performed segmentectomy 8 by a transfissural approach at that time. In this method, a surgeon can visualize the root of P8 in a fair operation field and success rate is above 80%. I would like to introduce a video.

First, the hilar Glissonean sheath is separated from the hilar plate. Right portal pedicle is encircled with a nelaton tube, and strangled to induce discoloration of the right lobe. The border is the main portal fissure. Then, parenchyma is transected using a CUSA or a Kelly clamp. The ventral part of the right portal fissure is dissected to expose the hilar plate so that the right anterior pedicle is visualized. At this point, the transection plane is tilted to the right side for approximately 2 centimeter, exposing the right surface of the P5(s) and P8(s). Vascular clamp is applied to the P8, and the segment 8 is discolored. The discolored liver surface is marked with Bovie. The transection of the main portal fissure continues in the depth where the MHV is exposed. A transverse parenchymal dissection to the right side in this depth is performed until the RHV is seen. At the meantime, the right border of the segment 8 is dissected following the anterior surface of the RHV. After segmentectomy 8 is complete, the cut surface is coagulated with bipolar coagulator and sealed with tachocomb and fibrin glue.

cf. Two videos about other approaches
Segmentectomy 8 part 2: Makuuchi technique (ICG dye injection)
Segmentectomy 8 part 3: Takasaki technique

7.13
Right anterior sectionectomy of anterior-dominant variant liver (Figures 31-33)

After laparotomy, adhesion from previous cholecystectomy is taken down. Right lobe of the liver is mobilized. Hilar Glissonean pedicles are lowered from the hilar plate, and right anterior and posterior pedicles are encircled separately with nelaton catheters. By temporary strangling of each pedicles, the border between the RAS and RPS is seen. As in the video, the temporary clamping of the right anterior pedicle discolors almost all parts of the right lobe saving a small portion of segment 6. This means that there is a variation in the intrahepatic vasculature of a anterior-dominant fashion. In another word, there might be one or more "sliding branch (es)" from the right anterior portal pedicle crossing the border to the RPS. To make an AR possible, first, the ventral main portal fissure is dissected to expose suprahilar Glissonean sheath. Then, the dissection continues to the right side to clear the right anterior pedicle from its root to the distal 1.5cm. At this point, a Glissonean pedicle branch that feeds RPS is seen. The right anterior pedicle distal to this branch is temporarily clamped and it discolored RAS territory similar to the livers with classic vascular structure. New right portal fissure is dissected along the demarcation plane. Then, the right anterior portal pedicle distal to the sliding branch is ligated, divided and sutured with 5-0 prolene. After completing the transection, the RAS is delivered out. As the video shows, the RHV and the MHV are exposed at the dissection plane.

7.14
Right anterior sectionectomy of posterior-dominant variant liver (Figures 35, 36)

After laparotomy, the liver was completely mobilized by taking down the ligaments. Cholecystectomy was performed. Initially a segmentectomy 8 was planned for this patient. Right pedicle was temporarily clamped to find the main portal fissure. Intraoperative ultrasound was performed to confirm the location of the tumor and relation to the MHV. The ventral portion of the main portal fissure was dissected. After dissection of the main portal fissure, small P8s were ligated and the liver surface was observed. Only a small portion of the segment 8 was discolored which did not include the tumor. Therefore, I additionally ligated few more branches that were thought to be feeding the segment 8, which, also, did not induce ischemia to the whole segment 8. A variation in intrahepatic vasculature where the Glissonean branches of the RPS crosses the border to the RAS territory was suspected. The plan was switched to perform a right anterior sectionectomy. The right anterior portal pedicle was temporarily clamped. In the video, you can see that only a small part of the RAS was discolored, and the tumor was seated beyond the discolored territory. This confirms that there is a sliding branch from the RPS to the RAS. First, the right anterior portal pedicle was ligated and divided. The parenchymal transection plane was, then, tilted to the right side, exposing the left surface of the right posterior pedicle. After clearing 2cm length of right posterior portal pedicle, a sliding branch that crosses the border to RAS was seen. This branch was ligated, and the segment 8 area was additionally discolored. The demarcation plane or a new right portal fissure was dissected and the RAS was delivered out.

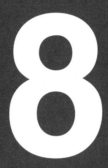

8

Tailored hepatectomy under the preoperative
3D image analyses: Tailored segmentectomy 8

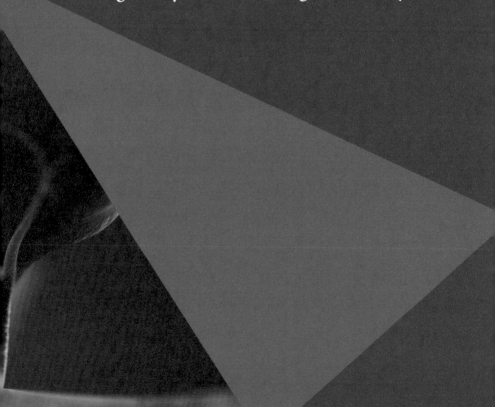

8

Tailored hepatectomy under the preoperative 3D image analyses: Tailored segmentectomy 8 (Figure 12, 13)

I want to discuss the tailored hepatectomy through the examples of various Glisson approaches of segmentectomy 8 in this chapter. Because we could get synapse 3D (Fuji film) in 2016, I could not know preoperatively the exact anatomical variation of third order branches in portal pedicle before 2016. At that time, the success rate of AR of segmentectomy 8 using Makuuchi procedure was relatively low, and that of Takasaki procedure was somewhat high. And its rate of transfissural approach was so high (more than 80%). From this reason, I had always chosen transfissural approach in segmentectomy 8 (Figure 54).

However, it has been possible for us to confirm the exact anatomical variation of third order branches of portal pedicle in preoperative simulation using Synapse 3D after 2016. Thereafter, I started the tailored hepatectomy according to the 4 types of anatomical variation of anterior portal pedicle in segmentectomy 8. I think it is desirable to choose a technique that is less invasive if possible. In terms of invasiveness, transfissural approach is the most invasive, followed by Takasaki technique and Makuuchi technique. Generally, I chose Makuuchi procedure for type A, Takasaki procedure for type B and C, and transfissural approach when type D or synapse 3D was not available. And, when Makuuchi technique failed, it was converted to Takasaki technique, and when Takasaki technique failed, it was converted to the transfissural approach **(Figure 55)**. Then, let's take a closer look at this selection process.

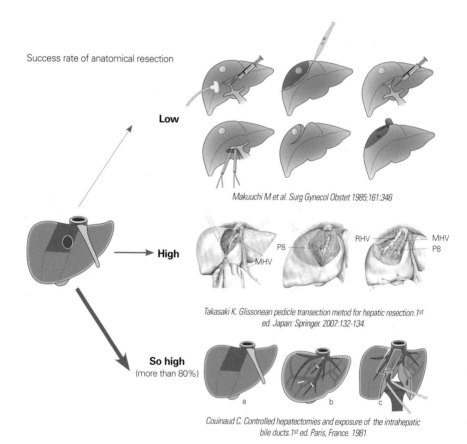

Success rate of anatomical resection

Low

Makuuchi M et al. Surg Gynecol Obstet 1985;161:346

High

Takasaki K. Glissonean pedicle transection metod for hepatic resection. 1st ed. Japan: Springer. 2007:132-134.

So high
(more than 80%)

Couinaud C. Controlled hepatectomies and exposure of the intrahepatic bile ducts. 1st ed. Paris, France. 1981

- **Figure 54   Before 2016: Era without 3D image**

My clinic could get the 3D image analyser (Synapse 3D, Fuji film) in 2016.
Therefore, we cannot analyze its 3D image preoperatively.
At that time, the success rate of anatomical resection for segmentectomy 8 was relatively low.
If I tried Makuuchi technique, its success rate was low, and if Takasaki technique, its rate was somewhat high.
However, if I applied transfissural technique, its success rate was more than 80%.

According to patterns of intrahepatic anatomical variation

Tailored approach

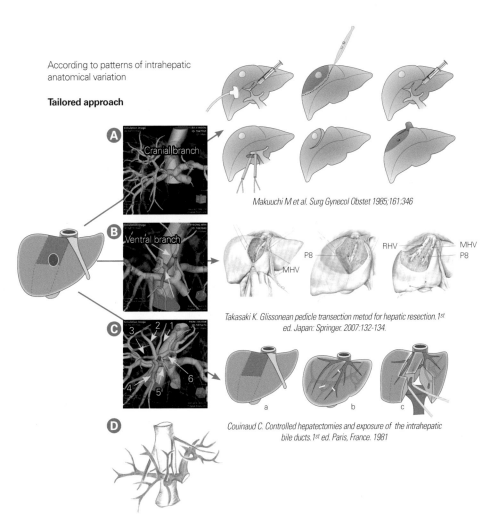

Makuuchi M et al. Surg Gynecol Obstet 1985;161:346

Takasaki K. Glissonean pedicle transection metod for hepatic resection. 1st ed. Japan: Springer. 2007:132-134.

Couinaud C. Controlled hepatectomies and exposure of the intrahepatic bile ducts. 1st ed. Paris, France. 1981

• **Figure 55   After 2016: Era with 3D image**

After 2016, we could apply a tailored approach in hepatectomy using preoperative Synapse 3D.
In type A, we applied Makuuchi's approach, and we chose Takasaki technique in type B.
And we performed "Transfissural approach" in type C, type D or not available state of preoperative 3D image.

8.1
Type A branching pattern of RAS on preoperative 3D image analysis

Type A: cranial-caudal type (49 cases, 46.2%)
The 3rd order portal branch of anterior portal pedicle have two or more branch and they go to the cranial-caudal direction.

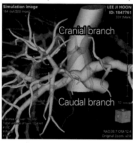
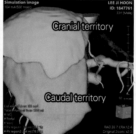
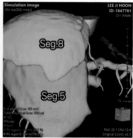

In type A RAS portal pedicle anatomy, two approaches can be undertaken. First approach is known as Makuuchi's method, whereby ultrasound-guided indocyanine green dye injection to a single P8 is performed to cause liver surface staining of segment 8. Cantlie's line and a transverse liver transection along the demarcation line is the first step to find a single P8. P8 is ligated and divided afterwards, and liver parenchymal transection is continued exposing the ventral portion of the RHV. A specimen containing segment 8, then, can be taken out after completion of liver dissection to the IVC at the superior border **(Figure 4)**. When P8 puncture is unpliant, or P8 branches are two or three, a second method can be attempted. This method is known as Takasaki's approach. In this procedure, the main right portal pedicle is temporarily clamped to induce ischemic demarcation to the right hemiliver. The cranial half of the demarcation line is dissected, and the P8 is, then, detected, ligated and divided at its root. Ischemic demarcation of segment 8 can be seen and process afterwards is identical to Makuuchi's method. The difference between two procedures is that the operator can see the anterior and right border of the segment 8 before liver parenchymal transection in Makuuchi's method, whereas in Takasaki's method, only its left border can be noticed before commencing the liver transection. If 3D images are available, given that there is only one P8, two method are equally simple and feasible.

cf. two videos
Segmentectomy 8 part 2: Makuuchi technique (ICG dye injection)
Segmentectomy 8 part 3: Takasaki technique

8.2
Type B or C branching type of RAS on preoperative 3D image analysis

Type B: ventral-dorsal type (14 cases, 13.2%)
The 3rd order portal branch of anterior portal pedicle have two or more branch and they go to the ventral-dorsal direction.

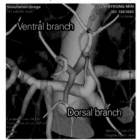
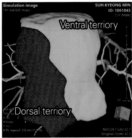
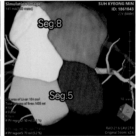

In type B RAS branching pattern, the third order branches of the right anterior portal vein spreads in ventral-dorsal direction. The P8s are consist of two or more fourth order branches arising from ventral and dorsal third order branches. In such cases, the success rate of Makuuchi's approach is very low. Takasaki's approach, in return, is preferred. The right portal pedicle is temporarily clamped and the cranial half of the main portal fissure is dissected along the ischemic demarcation line. The ventral branch of the anterior section is, then, confirmed, and the liver parenchymal transection is continued posteriorly to find superior 4th order branches toward segment 8. After they are ligated and divided, parenchymal dissection is more deepen posteriorly to find the dorsal branch of the anterior pedicle. Thereafter, if its superior 4th order branches toward segment 8 are also found, ligated and

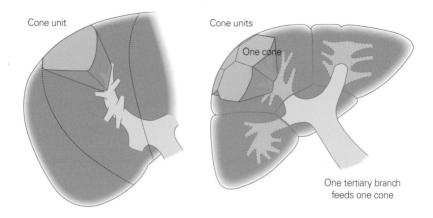

Cone unit

Cone units

One cone

One tertiary branch
feeds one cone

• **Figure 56   Cone unit concept of professor Takasaki.** [17)]

divided, segment 8 parenchyma is discolored and the operator can complete segmentectomy 8. It is a controversy, however, whether performing a segmentectomy by ligating multiple fourth order branches can be called an anatomical resection. And if ventral cone unit of RAS can contain the tumor, resecting the territory of the corresponding third order branch can be a more ideal approach as an anatomical resection. **(Figure 56)**

Cf. one video
Ventral cone unit resection of segment 8 in ventral-dorsal type of
portal Pedicles

Type C: Radial type (37 cases, 34.9%)
The 3rd order portal branch of anterior portal pedicle have multiple branches and they go to the radial direction.

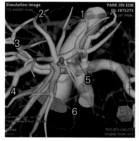
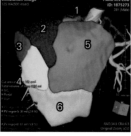
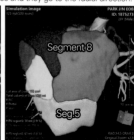

In case of irregular branching (more than 4) of the third order branches or type C branching pattern of RAS, segmentectomy 8 can be a challenge. Makuuchi's approach is not recommended. Likewise, liver parenchymal transection can be carried out by finding, ligating and dividing multiple P8s one by one using Takasaki approach. Since, it is not likely to be able to ligate all P8s at their roots, the success rate of anatomical resection is low. If the operator is determined to perform an anatomical resection, transfissural approach can be used as an alternative. As a first step, the hilar plate is lowered by blunt dissection, and right Glissonian pedicle is encircled with a nelaton tube. The ischemic demarcation of the right hemiliver can be observed by temporary clamping. Demarcation line is the main portal fissure. Then, transection of the liver parenchyma through the main portal fissure using CUSA or a Kelly clamp crushing is carried out until the dissection reaches hilar plate. Afterwards, the dissection plane is tilted to the right side exposing the left surface of the right anterior portal pedicle to find P5 and P8 within 2cm from the hilar plate. Temporary clamping of potential P8 branches may allow to visualize the segment 8 discolored territory at the liver surface. The ischemic anterior border of the discolored territory of the segment 8 is marked at the surface using Bovie coagulator. Parenchymal transection is continued toward the right side detecting segment 8 glissonean pedicles one by one until RHV is exposed. Following the RHV the dissection proceeds to suprahepatic IVC. Meanwhile, dissection of the connective tissue to the right-hand side of the anterior surface of the IVC allows visualization of RHV trunk. An additional parenchymal dissection parallel to the RHV separates segment 8 from the liver. After extraction of the specimen, the cut-surface of the liver is coagulated with argon beam laser or a bipolar coagulator. Surgeon, then, finishes the procedure by reassuring hemostasis with Tachocomb seal or Fibrin glue spray.

8.3
Type D branching type (sliding of origin variation) of RAS on preoperative 3D image analysis

Type D: The right anterior Glission pedicles have slidden branch to/from posterior branch (6 cases, 5.7%) branch of anterior portal pedicle comes from posterior portal pedicle.

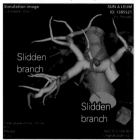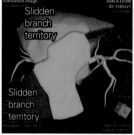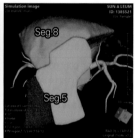

Anatomical resection is rarely achievable in type D variant anatomy of the RAS. A wedge resection is rather convenient. However, Takasaki's procedure or transfussural approach can be applied in case of anterior section dominant type. Contrariwise, in case of posterior section dominant type, wedge resection is preferred unless small contracted segment 8 can confine a small tumor.

8.4
Preoperative 3D image not available

Using 2-dimentional study only, limits the success rate of Makuuchi's procedure when conducting anatomical resection. Also, unawareness of P8's anatomical variation may consume excess amount of parenchymal dissection in order to find the root of P8 when attempting Takasaki's procedure. A considerable amount of hemorrhage can result since hemostasis is difficult. Even so, the success rate of anatomical resection is still low. At the time when 3D image was not available in our institution, I managed to perform segmentectomy 8 by a transfissural approach with a success rate of 80%.

This approach allows the visualization of P8 root in most of the cases, but it is an invasive procedure. The detailed procedure is described in section 6.1 and 7.2 **(Figure 52, 53)**, and a video: segmentectomy 8 part 1 (transfissural).

Anatomical Liver Resection
: Toward Tailored Surgery

9

Summary

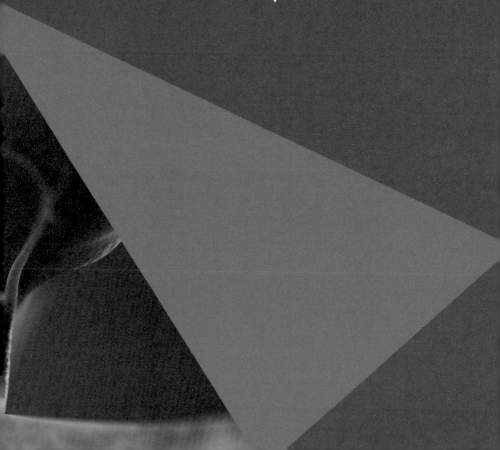

9

Summary

Hepatectomy is comprised of many steps of techniques. It is very difficult to discuss the superiority among various techniques of hepatectomy. In the evaluation of the superiority of hepatectomy techniques, the expertise and familiarity of the liver surgeons of each medical institution as well as the advantages of each techniques are critical. However, the most ideal hepatectomy techniques that is considered to be common among all surgeons are first, all types of hepatectomy must be systematically and universally applicable; second, the technique must be an effective so that the goal of the surgery is adequately accomplished; third, the procedure should be simple and easy; and last, the surgery must be performed safely despite anatomical variation. I discussed one of the hepatectomy techniques, focusing on the glissonean pedicle approach.

Couinaud stated that there are three approaches to the systematic hepatectomy technique. The first is the classical approach splitting the hepatic artery, portal vein and bile duct through the hilus. Then the each corresponding branches for the intended hepatectomy are confirmed, ligated, and divided, after which the stained liver parenchyme is excised. The second approach is the extrafascial approach, outside the Glisson sheath, in which hilar portal pedicle is detached from the hilar plate. And then pulling the Glisson pedicle to the inferior and contralateral direction, the 1st order and 2nd order branches can be identified. And then corresponding Glisson pedicle branches for the expected hepatectomy are confirmed and ligated, followed by removal of the stained liver. The third approach is opening the plane of the portal fissure, approaching through the fissure. Since the anterior liver is thin and thus easily exposed, the hepatotomy requires a little efforts, followed by confirmation, ligation and division of the corresponding Glisson pedicle branches for the intended hepatectomy. I used to utilize a complimentary approach of the above three methods according to the specific diseases or requirements.

In primary liver cancer patients, the extrafascial approach or transfissural approach is utilized. After the corresponding branches of the Glisson pedicle of the expected hepatectomy are confirmed and ligated, the stained liver parenchyme is resected. For hepatectomy in patients with Klatskin tumors or in donor and recipient of liver transplantation, the classical approach through the hilus is preferred, which consists of confirmation, ligation and division of the hepatic artery, portal vein and bile duct, respectively, followed by resection of the stained liver parenchyme.

Advantages of the glissonean pedicle approach in hepatectomy for hepatoma are that first, limited liver resection such as one segment resection is also permitted to systematic resection. Second, in hepatoma patients with accompanying liver cirrhosis, the portal venous collaterals or the engorged lymphatics within the Glisson sheath of the hepatic hilus are not disturbed during hepatectomy, which leads to minimizing of postoperative complications such as ascites. The third, even if an anatomical variation of the vascular pedicle of the liver is present during hepatectomy, complications such as inadequate injury of the vascular structures are also minimized.

If a hilar plate and umbilical plate is employed during the glissonean pedicle approach, the exposure of the Glisson pedicle is relatively facilitated, and the extrafascial approach is usually adequate for the resection of right and left liver or segment 2, 3, 4, 2+3 or 3+4b. However, it is not always possible in right side hepatectomies. Therefore, my main technique employed is hepatotomy through the anterior liver for the openings of the main portal fissure, umbilical fissure, and right portal fissure, followed by the glissonean pedicle approach within the liver. This method allows direct intraoperative identification of the many branches of the Glisson pedicle, which permits easy and accurate systematic hepatectomy by the operator.

Post-procedural liver function tests such as liver enzymes and total bilirubin levels after successful systematic liver resection are almost within the near-normal range. In contrast, non-anatomical resection such as enucleation or wedge resection results in long term abnormal liver function test. This is probably due to a remnant liver with an injured vascular pedicle. As described previously for systematic hepatectomy, there are various approaches for identifying the vascular pedicles. The evaluation of the superiority among these techniques is not desirable, because operator's choice and familiarity are very important factors in the treatment results of liver resection. If the reserved power of each individual medical institution permits, the technique that is simple, safe, and objective should be pursued.

Recent advances in 3D image technique and Professor Majno's three level of complexity theory have made possible to overcome the limitation of sixty-year old Couinaud's anatomical scheme. (Fig. 15) In summary, I dare to argue that the era of tailored hepatectomy whereby surgeons can apply different surgical approaches according to the patients' individual intrahepatic vascular variation.

10

Novel anatomy model of the liver and tailored hepatectomy

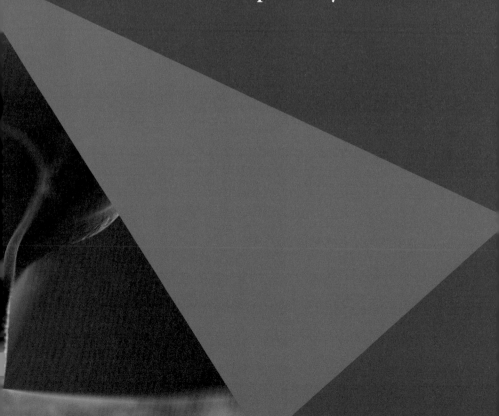

10
Novel anatomy model of the liver and tailored hepatectomy

So far, I have summarized the anatomy and the AR of the liver which I have experienced under Couinaud's dogma for 25 years. Nevertheless, Couinaud's theory which was created in the 1950s, has been the mainstream of the liver anatomy for 60 years to date in the absence of proper imaging technique and surgical instruments.

Recently a 3-dimentional depiction of the liver has become possible **(Figure 16, 17)** and with the aid of such technical breakthrough, Majno brought up a new way of comprehending intrahepatic vascular anatomy as the "1-2-20 concept". It is based on their observation of the intrahepatic vasculature such that the hepatic inflow or portal vein gives three 1st order branches; left, right anterior and right posterior; and further divides into random 2nd order branches, 9 to 44 in number (mean=20) rather than eight segmental branches, as conventional Couinaud's model describes **(Figure 14)**.[15] The notorious professor Henri Bismuth supported this view of liver anatomy and wrote in his editorial: "The paper by Majno et al. makes the interesting proposal that we should retain the Couinaud's division of the liver into 8 segments but that we should be ready to break free from it when, as radiologists and surgeons, we perform the complex procedures that the modern treatment of surgical liver disease requires.[16] It is indeed a new era of the "tailored hepatectomy".

As I reviewed this theory, I applied it to the Takasaki's cone unit theory which he wrote in his literature. The cone unit theory describes that the 2nd order branches of the Glissonean pedicle which feed the liver parenchyma from their root to the liver surface are irregular in number and in their way of branching (**Figure 56**).[17] Therefore, only left lobectomy, right anterior sectionectomy and right posterior sectionectomy that resect the feeding area of 1st order branches can be regarded as the AR, whereas other smaller resections are non-AR but rather are "cone unit resections" (**Figure 57**).

Takasaki's theory is parallel to Majno's, although the terminology is defined differently. Majno suggested the necessity of tailored hepatectomy based on

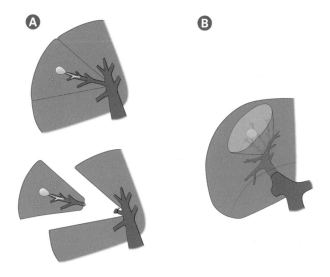

• **Figure 57** **Cone unit resection of professor Takasaki.**[17]
A. one cone unit resection. B. three cone unit resection.

the modern imaging analysis technology. Takasaki, likewise, described a novel anatomical theory and the techniques of hepatic resection.

In my experience of past 3 years, a high-resolution CT image that depicts minute 3rd order branches of the Glissonean pedicle (the same as 2nd order branches of Takasaki and Majno) is required in order to raise the success rate of ARs. I, also, found that the operative simulation using this 3D imaging prior to the surgery and confirmation of the resection territory with temporary ligation or dye staining technique during the surgery are crucial in navigative AR. This evidently proves that the hepatic resection under Majno's "second level of anatomy" is possible (Figure 15).

With the aid of the preoperative 3D imaging, contemplating diversion from AR to wedge resection (a non-AR) or from segmentectomy to lobectomy in anatomically variant liver can prevent an inadvertent intraoperative diversion while maintaining a high success rate of AR.

Lastly, in this new era of tailored hepatectomy, I would like to emphasize that the anatomical variation of the intrahepatic vasculature along with the baseline liver function must be taken into consideration before planning a hepatic resection.

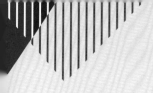

References

1. Korean J HBP Surgery 2011;15:101

2. Tajima T. et al. AJR 2002;178:885-897

3. Matsui O. et al. Imaging diagnosis of the liver. 1st ed. Tokyo, Japan: Igaku-Shoin. 1995:84-95

4. Miura K et al. Kan-Dan-Sui 2000;41:253-260

5. Makuuchi M et al. Surg Gynecol Obstet 1985;161:346-350

6. Billingsley KG et al. J Am Coll Surg 1998;187:471-481

7. Zhou Y et al. Langenbecks Arch Surg 2011;396:1109-1117

8. Chen J et al. Dig Dis Sci 2011;56:1626-1633

9. Torzilli G et al. Liver Cancer 2012;1:177-182

10. Suh KS. J Hepatobiliary Pancreat Surg 2005;12:365-370

11. Ishii M et al. World J Gastroenterol 2014; 20(12): 3335-3342

12. Sasaki K et al. The Am Surgeon 2013;79:1163-1170

13. Midorikawa Y, Takayama T. J Hepatobiliary Pancreat Sci 2012;19:48-53

14. Couinaud C. Controlled hepatectomies and exposure of the intrahepatic bile ducts. 1st ed. Paris, France

15. Majno P. et al. Anatomy of the liver: An outline with three levels of complexity – A further step towards tailored territorial liver resection. J Hepatol 2014;60:654-662

16. Bismuth H. A new look on liver anatomy: Needs and means to go beyond the Couinaud scheme. J Hepatol 2014;60:480-481

17. Takasaki K. Glissonean pedicle transection method for hepatic resection. 1st ed. Japan: Springer. 2007:25-26, 151-154

18. Wang HJ. Anatomical resection: Glissonean approach. 1st ed. Korea: Koonja Publishing Inc. 2015.

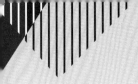

Index

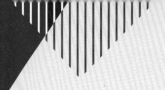